INTERMITTENT FASTING
for Women in their 40's & Beyond

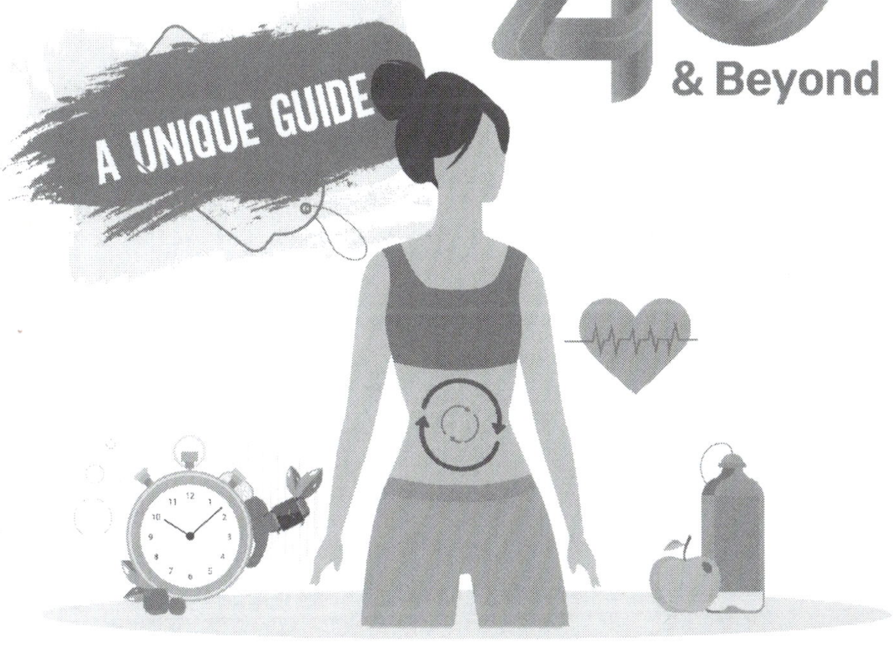

A UNIQUE GUIDE

WITH REAL-LIFE EXPERIENCES AND EFFECTIVE EXERCISES TO A HEALTHY WEIGHT LOSS AND LIFESTYLE WITHOUT STARVING OR DIETING

HOLLIS RICE

COPYRIGHT

Intermittent Fasting

for Women in their 40s and Beyond

By Hollis Rice

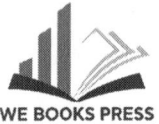
WE BOOKS PRESS

Copyright © 2021 We Books Press, New York.
All rights reserved.

No part of this publication may be copied, reproduced in any format, by any means, electronic or otherwise, without prior consent from the copyright owner and publisher of this book.

INTERMITTENT FASTING

DISCLAIMER

The information contained in this book is for general information purposes only. The information is provided by the authors and while we endeavor to keep the information up to date and correct, we make no representations or warranties of any kind, express or implied, about the completeness, accuracy, reliability, suitability or availability with respect to the book or the information, products, services, or related graphics contained in the book for any purpose. Any reliance you place on such information is therefore strictly at your own risk.

The author reserves the right to make any changes she deems necessary to future versions of the publication to ensure its accuracy.

INTERMITTENT FASTING

Table of Contents

Where it all Began — 7

Introduction — 8

CHAPTER - 01 11

The Physician Within — 11
What you need to know about Fasting? — 16
Your Choice of Fasting Techniques — 20
The Fasting Technique Relative to Different Time-Periods — 24
Why Should You Fast? — 27
Things You Should Expect When Fasting — 30
Factors Influencing Weight — 33
Why Do Some Diets Fail? — 36
The Medical Effects of Fasting — 38

Intermittent Fasting — 41

CHAPTER - 02 42

What is Intermittent Fasting? — 42
The 5 Goals of Intermittent Fasting — 44
Sacrifices That Comes with Intermittent Fasting — 47
Intermittent Fasting Vs Conventional Fasting — 49
Your Weight-loss Journey with Intermittent Fasting — 54
The First Changes You Notice — 58
The Body Balance — 60
More facts about Intermittent Fasting — 66

INTERMITTENT FASTING

CHAPTER - 03	70
The health benefits of Intermittent Fasting	70
The Healing Power of Fasting In The Mind & Body	72
Fasting and Anti-aging	75
Does Your Body Detox When You Fast?	78
Fasting & Fighting: The Battle with Addiction	81

CHAPTER - 04	86
Who can practice Intermittent Fasting?	86
Why Should You Practice Intermittent Fasting?	90
6 Reasons Intermittent Fasting Is Not for You	94
The Possible Health Risks	99

When to Eat — 103

CHAPTER - 05	104
When should you eat?	104
Your guide to Time-Restricted Eating	108
Why should you practice Time Restricted Eating?	110
Proven benefits of Time Restricted Eating	112
Practicing Time Restricted Eating	115

CHAPTER - 06	117
The Fast Diet –5:2 Diet Plan	117
Let's Start the 5:2 Diet	119
The Exact Way of Eating on Fasting Day	121
ALERT: Controlling the Overwhelming Hunger	123

CHAPTER - 07	125
The alternate-day fasting & 24 hours fasting	125
Essentials of Alternate-Day Fasting	127
Alternate Day Fasting and Hunger	129
Is Alternate Day Fasting Safe for People with Normal Weight?	132
What Happens in a 24 Hours Fasting?	134

INTERMITTENT FASTING

CHAPTER - 08 .... **136**

Clean Fasting Vs Dirty Fasting 136
Should I choose Clean Fasting? 139
Which one is the best? 144
The Verdict! 147

Tips & Tricks Just For You!   149

CHAPTER - 09 .... **150**

Why is Consistency and Physical Exercises are important in your
Weight-Loss Journey? 150
Physical Exercises 154
Exercise Suitable for Women Over 40 years 155
4 Easy Home Workouts to Burn Fat 161
Converting Outdoor Activities to Physical Exercises 164
5 Healthy Diet Recipes you must TRY! 166

The Proven Weight-Loss Journey   177

CHAPTER - 10 .... **178**

Real-Life Weight Loss Experience for Women over 40 years through
Intermittent Fasting 178
6 Celebrities Who Practice Intermittent Fasting 181

The Author's Point of View   182

Conclusion   186

References   189

Part

01

Where it all Began

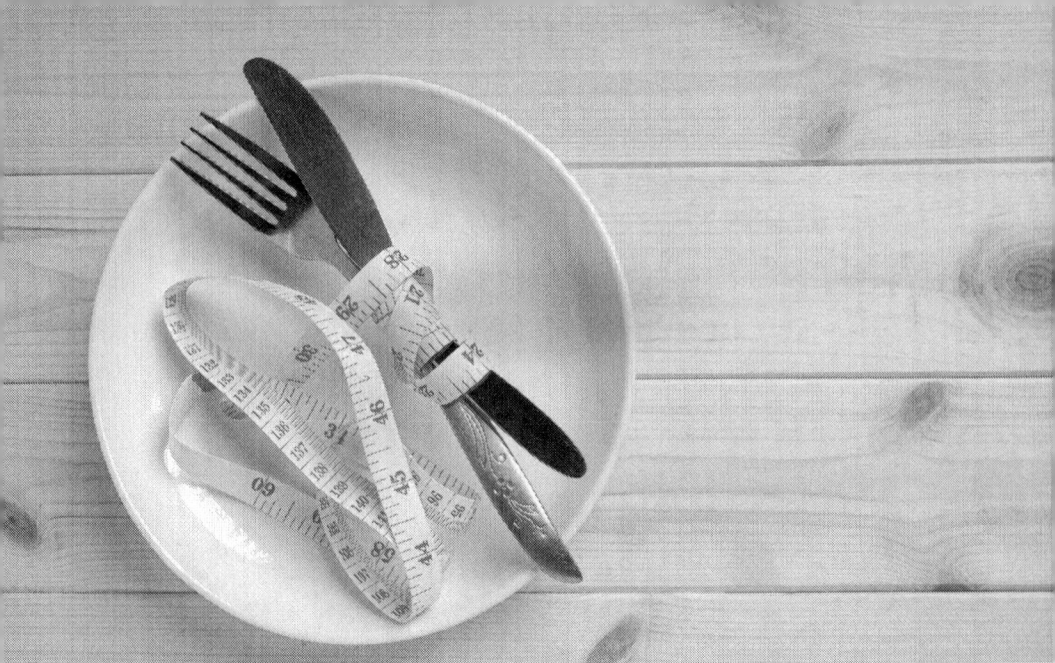

Introduction

Is your current diet not working anymore? Are you looking for effective ways to fast? Believe me the answers you have been looking for are right here in this book! Intermittent Fasting is not about starving yourself. You can consider yourself lucky, because in this book we will guide you in your weight-loss journey through the benefits of intermittent fasting including effective exercises suitable for women over 40's and best diet recipes you should try! This book has been written with references and sources which have all been verified and confirmed as reliable.

Intermittent fasting is a proven method for healthier living, and because it comes highly recommended for everyone but in this series, we will focus on women aged 40 years and above. Just like what they said: 'Life starts at 40'. You don't have to be an expert to fully understand this; we've made it easy for you!

INTERMITTENT FASTING

In the formative years of every single human being, knowledge, or the acquisition of knowledge is something that is seen as important. That is why we have so many levels in the education system, with each one of them bringing a new thing to the table via an increased workload- and helping to improve on the things that have already been learned at prior levels. This forms the fundamentals for acquiring knowledge.

However, it is also very easy to gloss over certain aspects of education and knowledge. What this means is that a few concepts seem commonplace, but when asked to explain in-depth, problems occur. One of these concepts is fasting.

Nine out of ten people will readily give you a definition of what they think fasting is and this is because the idea of fasting is far from being a new concept. The definitions may differ of course, as is the case with most things, but it is still known widely. For those who have a thirst for knowledge, and those who are willing to go ahead and put in the extra effort into learning, that is where this book comes in.

This book can be seen as a guide of sorts to understand what fasting is. You could count yourself as lucky to find such a treasure that is willing to answer your question as you present them. A very long period has been set aside to create this as a way of delving into what it means to fast and, perhaps more importantly, what intermittent fasting means.

For a topic as this one, a simple online search, or something as common as asking around will not be enough to answer the questions that an avid reader and knowledge seeker might have on this particular topic. That is why this book has been written with references and sources which have all been verified and confirmed as reliable. It is also important to note that this research encompasses the daily lives of individuals, and also takes into consideration the common misconceptions that people might have. It is an assurance that at

INTERMITTENT FASTING

the end of this book, all the questions that you might have with regards to any areas that pertain to fasting and intermittent fasting will be answered.

For those who have picked up this text without any prior knowledge of intermittent fasting, do not to worry. This will also for sure pique your interest.

Intermittent fasting is a proven method for a healthier living and because of that, it comes highly recommended for everyone. However, this book will mainly focus on the benefits of intermittent fasting for women in the age range of 40 years and above, although people who are not in this demographic can still benefit from its content.

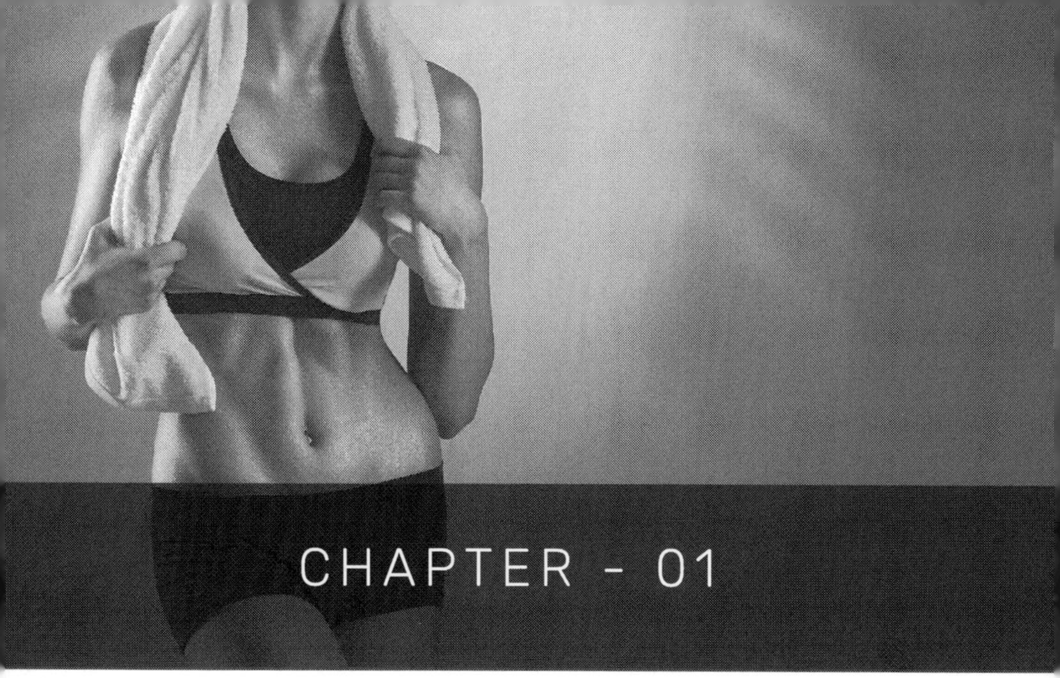

CHAPTER - 01

The Physician Within

Fasting is the greatest remedy --
the physician within.

PARACEISUS

A constant that has been in existence since the dawn of time, is the continual want for good things in life. We want to get a better job, we want to be paid more money, we want to have a comfortable life and more importantly, we want to live happy and healthy lives. The latter could have led to the concept of fasting.

INTERMITTENT FASTING

No matter what is or has been said, the need to feel good and better our lives has led to many inventions over the years which have and continues to help us all in every aspect of our lives. A good example of this is the leap in modern medicine and techniques. From the days of prodding through the skulls of patients to see what was ailing them, now that dangerous process is a lot safer and effective with the modern tools which can ensure a patient's higher rate of survival. This is aided by the modern equipment which can help in disease diagnosis without the need for a surgery.

Inventions like this, of course, have come from era to era, with tweaks and fine-tuning coming along the way as the idea moves forward. It is amazing to note that one of the longest-running practices that have been consistently used in a whole lot of different areas of daily life is fasting. It has been used in medical practices that date back to the 4th century, and has been a mainstay in religion and religious practices for far longer than that, even dating to the beginning of humans before any sort of organized civilization.

This shows that the practice of fasting has been tested and proven to work over the years. With the knowledge we have today, combined with all the additions and tweaking that have come into play over the years, the benefits of fasting have been studied intently and the fact that it is still being practiced today shows that it works.

I mentioned earlier that most of you would be able to give a simple definition of fasting and more often than not, that definition is; **"fasting is merely the abstinence of food".** This definition is not wrong in itself, but as you will come to see, there is a lot more to it than this and in order to get a clear picture, it would be best to look at the history of the fasting concept.

The earliest known jobs were those of the hunters and gatherers. While some went out to hunt wild animals for food, which was certainly more dangerous, others were tasked with gathering essentials like fruits, herbs and berries. By then it was long established that food was essential for life and as such, jobs were created to enable people provide food.

However, it should also be noted that this came way before the advent of organized agriculture when there weren't any stable sources of food. In early days, there were no farmers to plant food or rear animals for consumption, and as a result it was more than likely for people to go for long periods without having anything to eat. When the meals were eventually gotten, it would lead to cause for celebration, which in turn left us stuck with a *fast and feast* mentality and it can explain why it is biologically beneficial to fast. This, of course, is **Involuntary Fasting** it's still a concept that exists even today, although in a much different form and as a result of entirely different circumstances. Now you know just how deeply rooted this concept is, but let us now focus on **Voluntary Fasting.**

For a good example of voluntary fasting, you need not look any further than the ancient Greeks. They were one of the most advanced civilizations of their time. They made unimaginable leaps in medicine, the sciences and the arts. They were also great thinkers who knew that there was more to life and living than what meets the eye. Before the Olympic Games, athletes were known to fast for better stamina and strength as they prepared for the competition. It was very sacred that people would prove their seriousness to an oath by undergoing a fast.

A lot of scholars in the days of the Greeks felt like fasting would open their minds. It was seen as a "freeing of the mind" with the intent of learning more. A great example of this was Pythagoras, the world-famous Mathematician whose impact is still felt to this day, and his influence cannot be denied, as much of our understanding of mathematics is based on his research and reasoning.

A lesser-known fact about this great mind is that he tried to get into the prestigious Alexandria School in Egypt to learn more. He was however not able

INTERMITTENT FASTING

to, up until he fasted for forty days before he was able to take the exam and get into the school. This stands as a testament to how strongly one of the greatest minds to ever walk the earth felt about fasting. Other Greek physicians who believed in fasting are Plato and Hippocrates.

Plato professed love for fasting while stating that it provides mental and health benefits. This ideology and belief was carried on by his students, one of whom was Aristotle, who also expressed how important fasting was to him.

Hippocrates, who is widely regarded as the father of medicine believed in the benefits of fasting for longevity and good health. He was one of the first to propose that there was an "internal doctor" of sorts and that fasting was essential for its functioning.

Albeit the Greeks are just one example there are others too who believed in fasting. Egyptians for example, fasting was a norm, as we have already established from the story of Pythagoras' quest for knowledge. Most Egyptians were known to fast at least 30 times a year and this was deeply rooted in their societal and cultural beliefs.

The ancient Egyptians believed in moderation that could also benefit nature as well as themselves. They would embark on a fast because they believed that the restraint that they showed for such an essential thing in their lives would help them learn how to live without other excesses.

Fasting was and is also heavily featured in religion, religious rites and practices. It is widely preached and encouraged, with designated days set aside for fasting in Christianity during Easter celebration and in Islam in the month of Ramadan. Buddhists, in their pursuit of Nirvana, regard fasting as one of the major ways to stay unattached to the earthly distractions that hinder enlightenment.

Taoists in ancient China had a slightly different way of fasting or at least reasoning behind it. For them, it did not mean just staying without food instead, it was seen more along the lines of a practice that essentially feeds the spirit and not the body, unlike what eating would do. They used this as an essential step in the search for immortality. This concept moved on throughout history, with fasting being of a major significance to every civilization that rose, even up to slightly more modern eras.

Paracelsus, an alchemist, scholar and physician has been attributed to be one of the most important names in the Renaissance. He was one of the fathers of the medical revolution during this time. He said;

> Fasting is the greatest remedy—
> the physician within.

This is a call back to Plato's theory, that the body repairs and heals itself after a period of time. The only thing that is done to help this process is the lifestyles that we choose to acquire and add to it.

This is added to the unending list of people who have made a great impact during their lives, the lives of others and to the society at large. Fasting has also been used as a tool for change where there have been instances of protesters going without food for a certain period so that their voices can be heard. At this point, I am sure that I have proven without reasonable doubt that fasting is an essential and integral part of our lives and it's here to stay.

INTERMITTENT FASTING

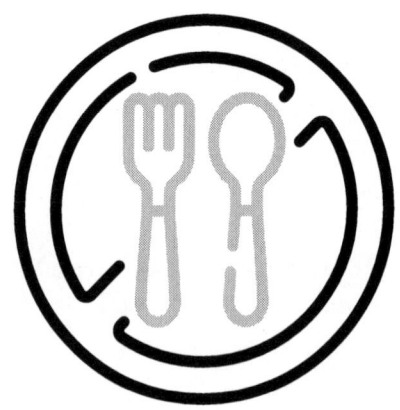

What you need to know about Fasting?

At this point, you have an idea about what fasting might mean. It has already been established earlier that its meaning may vary widely and may mean a lot of different things to different people. However, it would be remiss if a standard definition is not given, one that at least tries to encompass most of these different ideologies on the same topic.

For a standard definition, we will be considering one of the most widespread dictionaries in the world, the Oxford English Dictionary.

> noun. /f st/ /fæst/ a period during which you do not eat food, especially for religious or health reasonsto go on a fast - Fasting (Oxford English Dictionary).

INTERMITTENT FASTING

However, this is a standard definition, and for the next few decades, there might be no alterations to it of any sort. So, while it will stand for longer, it seems too rigid for such a fluid concept.

Right out of the gate, we see what is considered as one of the two main reasons to embark on a fast, that is religious and health reasons. It is important to note that this book will focus more on the latter, the main logic being that health is a more widespread and all-encompassing topic, while religion and religious practices may differ from person to person.

I took a small focus group recently, and when I asked them what fasting meant, most replied that they think fasting is staying away from food for a while. The interesting thing about this focus group is that, even though most of them were not particularly religious, or had any affiliation with a religious body, majority of them considered that a fast might be held based on religious beliefs, like the Buddhists who are known to embark on very long fasts

What was more interesting, was the fact that most people did not realize the health benefits of fasting and Sadly, this is because fasting has been played down over recent years, not because its health benefits have suddenly become lacking, but because the modern world and all the industries it comes with are constantly trying to sell you something. I will go into more detail on this below, as we deal with one of the first concepts that will be discussed in this book.

— THE FASTING-PROFIT DYNAMIC

At first glance, I am sure you considered that this might just be a concept for how much you profit from fasting but it is deeper than that.. Although it seems a bit complicated, trust me, you will understand in a minute.

I have hinted at the health benefits of fasting, which were hammered upon by our ancestors and scholars in the centuries prior to ours, but it seems like

INTERMITTENT FASTING

there has been a rapid decline in the public interest in fasting in recent years. This brings us to the question, why has the interest and knowledge of fasting declined so rapidly and abruptly? Well, the answer is simple, there is NO profit to be made!

We live in, arguably, the most consumer-driven period in history. You turn on the television and you are bombarded with ads and commercials that try to sell common things to you. You walk out of your house and you see these huge billboards with products that you had not considered at first, but they gradually begin to appeal to you. This is entirely intentional. It's important to know millions go into research things that people want or need, and then millions go into marketing those products to you.

You didn't know you wanted that new self-cleaning vacuum cleaner until you saw it the other day. You had not considered that new smart fridge until the ad came up after your soap opera. But where are the ads telling you to fast? Where are the commercials giving you advice on how to take care of yourself, without simultaneously trying to sell you something? There aren't any. This is because they cannot turn a profit unless there is something to sell, and you cannot sell fasting. Multi-billion-dollar food industries aren't going to tell you to take some time off their meals and take care of yourself. Instead, they'll sell you food that is supposed to help with weight, or they end up trying to invent new and healthier alternatives because there is profit to be made.

Another aspect of this is in the world of medicine it becomes an unending cycle. The food industry sells food that can lead to health problems, and the medical industry does not recommend fasting as their first line of defense. Instead they sell the medicine to fix this because there is profit to be made here as well As such we eat the poison, "food" and buy the cure, "medicine". But what is best for the consumer?

INTERMITTENT FASTING

The answer is "Fasting"! That is conscious abstinence from food for health reasons and longevity. It helps the physician within and it does its best to keep you healthy. This in turn helps you save money and as a bonus, you learn a measure of self-control, as the Egyptians figured out a very long time ago. The habit moves into other areas of your life, teaching you prudence and self-control.

So, now you understand the dynamics at play when it comes to fasting and profit. Fasting profits the individual, but the sale of products profits the businesses selling them. This contributes to the reduced knowledge of what fasting is and its importance in our daily lives. It is safe to say that this is a new concept for most of you reading this, and now that we have made it this far, it seems best to offer my congratulations.

Next, we'll go deeper into fasting, by considering a few techniques that could help you.

INTERMITTENT FASTING

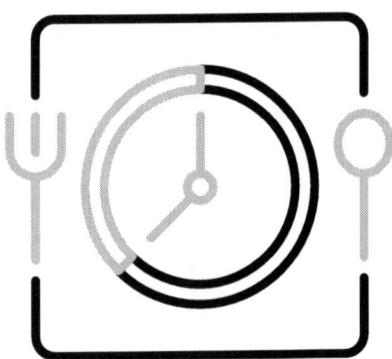

Your Choice of Fasting Techniques

So, you're learning about fasting, and you begin to wonder what are the various fasting options I can try? Well, that's where fasting techniques come into play.

Fasting techniques are essentially ways to fast it's really that simple. Of course, some ways are more difficult than others, and they may differ on a personal, religious, or even moral basis. To help you grasp this information better, I'll list out a few people and the types of fasting that they have embarked on. Please see below;

INTERMITTENT FASTING

— SELECTIVE FASTING

This form of fasting is done by almost everyone at some point in their lives, although it may not be voluntary. So, for the rest of this passage, we will discuss its voluntary aspects.

What is selective fasting? This simply means staying away from certain meals, food, or even entire food groups. An example of this was the ancient Greeks. We have already looked into a few key figures and their significance to the history of fasting. They would sometimes leave meals that they felt were unfavorable, especially in preparation for big events. Another example was the athletes who would leave our certain meals to prepare for the Olympic Games. That tradition is not out-of-place even today, as athletes from different places and those who participate in different sports still keep away from meals that will not help or maybe even hinder their progress. Although it is a debate that veganism and vegetarianism can be considered as types of selective fasts, it is more widely accepted to consider both things as separate concepts all on their own.

— THE FRUIT FAST

This is quite common but most people do not know that this is a type of fast. For the sake of this text, we won't consider those who embark on this type of fast involuntarily, but it is important to note that this brings the same result as most of those who voluntarily embark on this. However, things done with a full mind often yield better results because adhering to a schedule, or timetable and drawing up a meal plan works better in the long run than doing it haphazardly. An example of a historical person who embarked on a food fast was Adam and Eve. Even though this may be a sore spot for some, as this is a religious reference, it should be noted that it is their lifestyle story that should be taken into account. The first man and woman lived on a strictly fruit-based diet where they were told to eat from any tree in the garden, save one. This showed that their meal plan consisted only of fruits from trees since they did not eat any of the animals or animal products.

INTERMITTENT FASTING

However, this is just one example, as even today, there are many cultures and sects of people whose meal plan revolves around the sole consumption of fruits and without any other food. Fruits are good for your body, and even though this is not highly regarded, as it still involve consumption. The next fasting technique is a lot more common and well known to most people

— **THE WATER FAST**

Water is life. That's a saying that transcends time and people. No matter where you are, or who you are, you need water for survival. Even just a couple of hours without water can lead to early signs of dehydration. If you pair this with hot or even moderately warm weather, what you're left with is just utter disaster.

Water fast is a practice where an individual does not consume any food or drink other liquids than water. This is quite common, and even more widely considered as a form of fasting, even more so than fruit fasting. This is because the importance of water in our system cannot be over-emphasized. It is used in many body metabolic processes to be overlooked as merely something that can be done without. Examples of this type of fast are very common today and are not restricted by culture or religious practices, although some religions dictate a more hardcore form of fasting, and that form of fasting has been elaborated more, as you will see below. However, before that you should probably know that water fast is just one of the many different types of liquid fast, which involves the sole consumption of liquids and liquid food. An example of someone who lived like this was Angus Barbieri.

Angus Barbieri was a Scottish man who lived in the twentieth century, from 1939 to 1990. In 1965, he embarked on a liquid fast until July the following year. This fast lasted for a total of 382 days, an incredible feat! During this time, he only consumed liquids and at the very end of his fast, he had lost almost 280 pounds. He was recognized by the Guinness book of world records and the holder for the world record of the longest fast without solid food. Who knows? Maybe one of the readers of this book could beat that!

THE DRY FAST

So, you're at work and a colleague comes up to you and says, "Hey, I've been thinking and I think I'm going to go on a fast for a month." Usually, the first thing that pops into your head is how much of a long time that is to go without food or water. That image that you got is the very definition of a dry fast. A dry fast involves abstinence from any sort of food, in any form. This means no food and no water. As difficult as this may seem, this is the most recognized form of fasting. As shown earlier, this is what would come into any person's head at the mention of a fasting exercise.

A lot of people are turned off from it because it seems like a lot of work to do, but in most cases, it isn't. There is a reason why only good testimonies can be seen from undergoing such an endeavor. From those who talk about their tremendous weight loss to those who feel lighter mentally, to those who use it as an exercise to learn prudence.

I would like to emphasize that it is always best to exercise restraint and moderation in this in order not to hurt yourself, but lucky for you, this book will provide guidelines on just the right things to do.

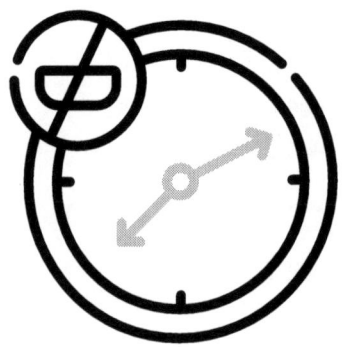

The Fasting Technique Relative to Different Time-Periods

We have touched on a lot of history so far and it's a good thing, since it shows that fasting is one of the few unchanged traditions that still exist to date. The ability to stay without food for certain periods does not seem like the sort of thing that would stand the test of time. The reason we keep going back into things that have happened in the past is to learn. We look at our history and see the ups and downs; we learn what created those ups while simultaneously learning not to recreate the event that led to the downs.

FASTING BEFORE ORGANIZED AGRICULTURE

As stated earlier although not in detail, the advent of organized agriculture put an end to a lot of habits. This was still a long time ago, but before the invention of farming and its organization, regular meals were not a thing.

INTERMITTENT FASTING

The concept of eating three times a day is a moderately new invention putting in consideration the entirety of human existence. For such a long time, meals were eaten when they were acquired. Early hunters would eat when they found animals that they could kill and eat. Early gatherers would eat when they found trees with fruits, berries, or other things like that.

Organized agriculture was the first stable source of food. It still had its downsides of course, but as is the same with each new idea, as years passed there were a lot more contributions to it. The inventions of new agricultural processes brought things like crop rotation, which helped the growth of crops all year round, leading to a continuous and steady supply of meals.

Before this, some studies have shown that even when meals were gotten, they would be kept and stored until certain hours in a day, when they would be eaten.

FASTING AFTER ORGANIZED AGRICULTURE

Nothing shows voluntary fasting like the abundance of food. The ability for self-control to be maintained in times of plenty shows the actual essence of the fasting exercise.

This helps to explain how important fasting became with the rise in mass production of food. Meals were readily available and refusing them helped to prove a point. While sometimes it was to prove a point, other times, it was to show remorse and/or to exercise self-control. Soon, the health benefits came to light and the process was shown to be as effective as some of the other solutions to weight loss.

It was during this time that fasting was more fine-tuned towards special methods that would be used for different events and reasons. Here, it became more choice-based and showed that people were willing to forgo certain things in life, not because they didn't have access to them, but because they chose to. Here, we can say that fasting increased significantly in importance. From this, the health benefits started to become clearer. For example, even though the Egyptians saw fasting as a prudence exercise, the Greeks looked at it more along the lines of health and its relation to it. That was why many great thinkers like Aristotle, Plato, and Socrates vouched for the powerful effects of fasting.

Another good example worth to note, which has been mentioned before is Hippocrates. The father of modern medicine was the first to talk about the physician within, which was the body's innate ability to repair itself. He also postulated that nothing helped this as much as fasting did. The myriad of examples that are there to pull from, gives a better understanding of the subject.

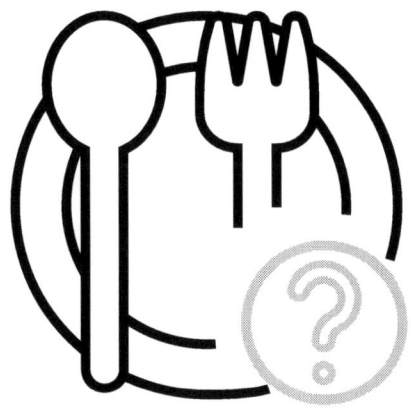

Why Should You Fast?

The reasons why people would want to embark on a fast are numerous. The reasons cover a far range, just like the reason why you are reading this book. For example, people might pick up this book because they need answers to it. Some might be going through these pages to learn more about the entire concept of fasting. Others might read this book because they are looking for a fitness plan to get healthy. Either way, all of these questions, however vast they are, have been answered in this book.

Just like those questions, the same goes for the reasons why people fast. They are incredibly numerous and each has its importance and significance. Of course, all of these reasons vary from person to person. For the sake of easy comprehension, we have consulted with a focus group within the age range of this book and through that, we have successfully gathered the major reasons why people embark on a fast. These reasons will be further explained in the next part of this text starting with the most common reason there is.

INTERMITTENT FASTING

— IT'S YOUR CHOICE

It is really that simple. The choice is the number one reason why people would embark on a voluntary fast. It's a lot less grand than other reasons, but this is the main reason. The idea of choice is the main thing that moves people to fast. It is the very concept behind voluntary fasting, and therefore it is the most popular. The ability to choose intrigues people, especially when there is something to lose and gain.

Most people who choose to fast have readied their mind to stay without food or water, depending on the fast that they have decided to do. It takes an incredible amount of self-control as does any other type of fast.

— THE PEER INFLUENCE

The role of a peer group should not be downplayed in the power to make people do things. Each one of us has friends or family around us, and if you think hard enough, you'll notice a few habits that you have adopted from them. Usually, since these are your friends, these habits are harmless. It can range from subtle things like copying their mannerisms and speech patterns to some larger things, like taking on a hobby of theirs, maybe a sport or an exercise.

Therefore, there are always things that can circulate to every member of a particular peer group. It might be why you have a spin class planned for next week, or why you have a magazine subscription that you always forget to cancel. It makes sense for an idea to spread around a peer group. This can be a way in which people adopt the culture of fasting.

— SOCIAL MEDIA

Most of what we take in and learn subconsciously comes from what we see around us. These days we aren't surrounded by trees and plain fields anymore.

Instead, we continue to be constantly barraged by these unending ads and commercials that show us what they think we need. A fact about this is that even if we don't exactly need these things, it doesn't change the fact that in the end, we are somehow convinced otherwise.

This can come with benefits of course and now the media can be a reason behind people's fasting. They may be made aware through articles and books such as this and then, they will learn what fasting is. This available medium, when used properly can act as a driving factor and as a reason why people decide to embark on fasts.

HEALTH AS THE PRIME REASON

This is the most common reason for a fast. A lot of research has been put into learning the effects of a fast and how it relates to health. We have already mentioned it in this book, with examples like the physician within and other topics which will further be explained later.

With that being said, it is only logical for people to want to fast for the health benefits. The ancient Greeks understood this and gave many testaments to the vitality they felt each time they embarked on a fast. It was seen as more of a way to cleanse the body of all the impurities that it possessed.

So, when people embark on fasts because of the medical benefits, they are not far from the truth. With advantages ranging from weight loss to cleansing, it is easy to see why this is done. It's perfectly normal to go on a fast for the benefits that it contributes to your health and wellbeing. It is also important to note that this has been well established for a long time because it fasting works!

INTERMITTENT FASTING

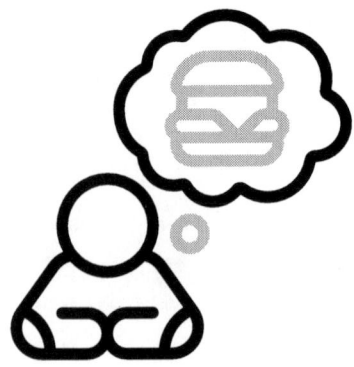

Things You Should Expect When Fasting

There is always expectation for results for everything that is done and this is true for most endeavors that we decide to accomplish. We already mentioned that we always want to be better, and most things can contribute to us being better and readily accepted. Because of this, anything that is not going to yield an outstanding result is often overlooked and overshadowed by things that have been proven to work time and time again. Fasting is one of those things that we now know works.

If you are the type of person that wants results, then it is normal to want to know what to expect from going on a fast and the following are just a few of the things you should expect when you fast.

INTERMITTENT FASTING

It is normal to feel hungry:

As simple as this may look, it is a common problem for people and the cause of misconceptions on the topic of fasting. The fact that other people have embarked on lengthy fasts does not mean that they do not feel hungry. All this shows is that they have toned themselves to be able to endure more. That is just like in any exercise routine, it is hard at first, but eventually, it becomes easier as you get used to it.

You will feel a strain:

For a body that is not used to something, it takes a while adapt to a new thing. This is how fasting feels especially if it's for the first time. There will be a strain on you, depending on what type of fast you do, and for how long you do it, but that's what this is for. Just by reading this, you will learn about how to pace yourself and see what is right for you.

Health Benefits:

For an exercise like fasting, the health benefits are not optional. The more fasting becomes consistent, the more the results start to show up as well. They go hand in hand. These health benefits include weight loss, improved immunity, and overall body fitness. These are a surety once you decide to fast.

Self-control:

It has been long said, and it is still iterated today that fasting is an exercise in self-control. It takes a lot to deprive yourself of a basic human necessity, but it is not impossible. Continuation of such an endeavor increases a person's accommodation for self-control. This ends up spilling into other areas of one's life, proving that there are certain things that we can indeed live without or at least handle in moderation.

INTERMITTENT FASTING

The above are just a few things to expect from fasting. Just like any exercise, it takes a while to get used to and it does not bring out results immediately. However, consistency will go a long way in helping and soon enough, with the right plan and schedule, it becomes part of your life. All these, as I've mentioned, require the appropriate type of fasting, one that is the subject of this book, and that is **Intermittent Fasting**. It more than encompasses all these areas in terms of results, health, and overall benefits.

Before we go into intermittent fasting as a topic, there are a few things that you should learn first, for a better understanding of the subject, such as body weight and dieting.

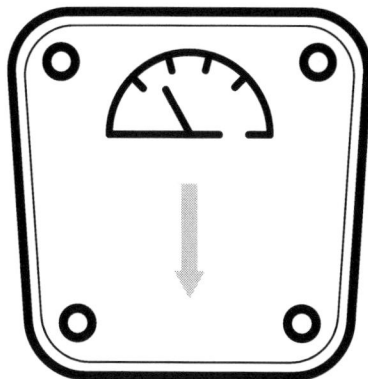

Factors Influencing Weight

A person's weight is a sensitive topic for most, and it is a tool used to market things to people. Most of these are things such as for gaining and losing weight end up falling flat, because they do not take the origin of a person's body weight into consideration.

Weight is mainly genetic. That is why there are people who can eat and drink whatever they want and yet they won't gain a single pound! We have people like that around us, and maybe you the reader of this book might be the same way, but this does not always equal to being healthy.

There is a group of people who are built in a way that makes it easy for them to gain weight, sometimes by not even trying. That is why knowledge of the specifics of genetic make-up is needed. It's good to take note of your body and its habits to understand and create what would work for you. That is why there are no specific ways to fast. Instead, there is a wide array of meal plans and guidelines for a fast. There are also different levels to this, for those with more or less endurance.

It is all-encompassing and therefore is a lot better than useless products which play to general insecurities which instead of trying to help with the problem, they only act as a reminder and in some bad cases, they act as reinforcements of the weight gain.

Genes are not the only factors, but they top the list. Other factors include;

1. Sex
2. Age
3. Sleep patterns
4. Eating habits
5. Physical activities
6. Culture
7. Medical conditions

BODY MASS INDEX

Body Mass Index or BMI is a metric that involves the use of weight and height to measure and screen people into the various weight categories. These categories are;

1. **Underweight:** The underweight category is characterized by having a BMI of below 18.5 when measured.
2. **Normal Weight:** This is the normal category and it is characterized by having a body mass index between the range of 18.5 - 24.9 when measured.
3. **Overweight:** Those who fit into the range of 25.0 - 29.9 are classified into the overweight category.

4. **Obese:** Obesity is extreme body fat, which is usually accompanied by health issues. This is characterized by people when their BMI is from 30.0 and above.

This method requires nothing more than a basic knowledge of math and a calculator. The calculation for this is the person's weight in kilograms divided by the square of their height in meters.

For example, for a person weighing 80kg with a height of 185cm (1.85m) the BMI calculation would be as follows;

$$80/(1.85)^2 = 23.4 \text{ (Normal Weight)}$$

This calculation serves to help any individual, not just to know the category they fit into, but also to know if they are on the brink of falling into another category. That helps to understand what plan would be essential for each person and what they need to work on. Those who fit into the extremes can use this to work towards their goals, and also track the progress that they have made so far. It should also be noted that falling into a category such as normal weight doesn't mean that you are healthy. You could fall into any of these categories and still have health issues.

INTERMITTENT FASTING

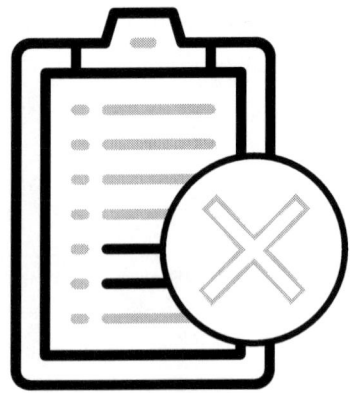

Why Do Some Diets Fail?

It's easy for anyone to suggest a diet to you. It's the most common thing that people think about when in a conversation about weight loss. Let's say you tell your friends that you want to lose some weight, the usual response or the thing that they would suggest is a diet, especially if physical exercise is not a ready option at the moment. The diet just seems easier, you know? A few snips to your meals and staying away from a couple of things that are supposed to be unhealthy, like junk food, soda, and sugar.

The question now is why do they fail? If diets are so common that they are the first thing for people to suggest, then why do they fail? Why are they now a laughing stock that no one takes seriously?

For more emphasis on this, notice how quick people are to throw away a diet. It is always riveting to start a new diet and eating guide. A lot of people have one diet or another planned out for themselves and in the end, after just a few days or weeks, they fall off the wagon. That's not always the case though. Sometimes people complete their diet, but just a few short days after that and they are back to their unhealthy selves. This ends up defeating the purpose of the entire thing in the first place.

It's a case that continues to happen over and over and that makes people wonder why diets fail, even when they are so advertised. The truth is, it's not just the fault of the diet itself, but diets alone aren't enough. Diets gives you a lifestyle for a short period, but the moment the dieting period is over, we go back to our habits that gave us health issues in the first place. This is where the self-control factor of fasting comes into play. Regular fasting helps you learn how to manage your hunger.

A region in the brain called hypothalamus is the centre for controlling a person's appetite and feeding behavior. It is responsible for the feelings of both hunger and satisfaction before and after a meal is consumed. In animals, when this is affected and the satiety center is destroyed, they lose their ability to feel full or satisfied after a meal and because of that they eat and eat (hyperplasia), leading to what is called hypothalamic obesity. The research however proves that the feeding and satiety center can be altered and trained by fasting.

Fasting helps you with hunger management. The planning and timing of meals help in training the satiety center on hunger patterns. Often, if you repeatedly do something, automatically you get used to it. Another advantage that fasting has over regular dieting and sometimes even exercise is just how inexpensive it is to do. All of these combined helps to push it ahead as the more appropriate thing to do.

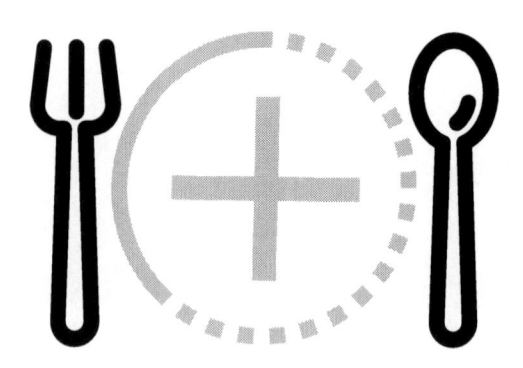

The Medical Effects of Fasting

A lot of benefits have been said to come from fasting and because of this a lot of research has also been put into finding its medical benefits. This has yielded good results over the years and the medical effects span a wide range of areas such as;

BLOOD PRESSURE

Fasting has been proven to have good effects in regulating blood pressure which helps to prevent heart complications. A study that involved 110 obese adults undergoing supervised fasting for three weeks proved this by showing significant reductions in blood triglycerides (by up to 32%) and LDL cholesterol (by up to 25%)

— BOOSTING BRAIN FUNCTION

An increase in brain function has been associated with the exercise of fasting. Research done has shown a correlation between improved brain health and scheduled fasting periods. This means increased cognitive function, with added help in brain structure and general health.

— WEIGHT LOSS

This deserves a chapter of its own. The benefits are tremendous. Most people can even pick fasting just so that they can shed a few pounds, but unlike starvation, fasting has added advantages. A review shows that whole-day fasting exercises can reduce weight by about 9%.

Part

02

Intermittent
Fasting

CHAPTER - 02

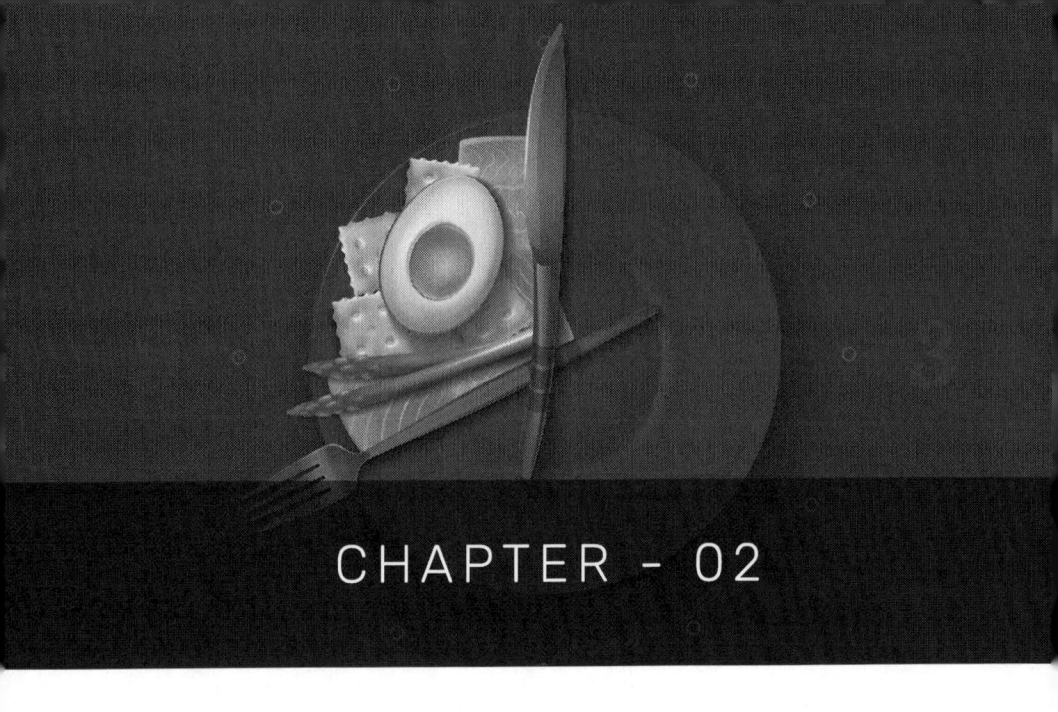

What is Intermittent Fasting?

It's almost impossible to discuss fasting in general without mentioning intermittent fasting. First it is important to note that intermittent fasting is not starving yourself. Intermittent fasting is intentional and is not involuntary like some of the techniques that we have already gone through.

Intermittent fasting means the pattern or cycle set in place between the periods of eating and fasting. What this means is that intermittent fasting is a set period of eating and a set period of fasting, all rolled into a timetable of sorts.

From this definition, it's easy to understand that we already do a sort of intermittent fasting by eating breakfast, lunch and dinner. This is technically true, but there are still no set times. Another example is when we are asleep and wake up. The whole concept of breakfast in the first place is to break the fast that was taken during sleep.

INTERMITTENT FASTING

There are various methods of doing this, but these are categorized based on certain times allocated to each period. There will be more on this later on.

It is important to note that intermittent fasting is not the same as fasting in general. It is easier to think about it with more focus directed towards the time of the meal, than what is eaten. In most cases, the meal doesn't matter and that's the major difference between fasting and dieting. Intermittent fasting is not bound by diet, so meal proportions and properties don't always have to be considered. However, this does not mean that food is not important. Also, you can't fast and then focus on junk food, because that would only counter the process. It just means that one is more important and that is the cycle.

Intermittent fasting is not a new invention though and it doesn't change from time to time, the way various diets do, but what it has been, is consistent. The methods to apply it are numerous, and that gives people a wide array of options to choose from. That way they can pick what is best tailored to fit them. There are many testaments of the wonders of intermittent fasting online from fitness experts to celebrities.

The 5 Goals of Intermittent Fasting

I know that most people have specific reasons for going on an intermittent fast. Maybe they want to feel better about themselves, or maybe they need a technique to help with their health. Either way, it is the right choice.

Intermittent fasting was designed to get a level of consistency in play, and that is one of the main things that will come up a lot in the following pages and chapters in this book. This need for consistency is the main reason behind the invention of fasting. Things should be done with a plan and an order in mind. This is intermittent fasting! It was invented to provide that stability.

Just like how exercises are measured in reps to provide a pattern to follow, that is exactly how intermittent fasting is to regular fasting. This is notably the best way to get that progress that we search for. The goals of intermittent fasting will be discussed in the next few headings.

REGULATION OF HORMONE CIRCULATION

When food isn't consumed for a while, the hormone production and circulation become even stronger as a result of the need for new nutrients. Intermittent fasting ends up being the signal that jump-starts this process. The regular timing and intervals help in the regulation until it becomes second nature.

The hormones that are circulated do so to release much-needed protein which is usually stored in the body. Examples of these hormones include; insulin, Human Growth Hormone (HGH), hormones for cellular repair, gene expression and many more.

REDUCTION OF INSULIN RESISTANCE

One of the most common health problems is the appearance of type 2 diabetes. It has become one of the most recurring diagnoses in recent years. Granted, this can be caused by genetic factors more often than not, but intermittent fasting can help, especially when there is a history of this in the genetic background.

The reduction of insulin resistance helps to also reduce the level of blood sugar in the blood. This in turn helps in protecting against type 2 diabetes. Studies show that intermittent fasting reduces insulin resistance and that is its correlation with type 2 diabetes.

ENSURING A HEALTHY HEART

The world's biggest killer currently is the heart disease. Cardiovascular diseases are responsible for more than 30% of the total deaths in the world. This is a result of several risk factors that almost anyone is prone to. Thankfully, one of the goals of intermittent fasting is to help with this. Intermittent fasting serves to improve these risk factors to help with a reduced chance of heart disease in the short and long run.

INTERMITTENT FASTING

— INDUCTION OF CELL REPAIR

Fasting could be seen as a resting state for the body. During this time, it is normal for worn out or damaged cells, and sometimes tissues to start to repair themselves. They do this through a process called autophagy, which is the removal of waste.

Increased autophagy by cells has been proven to lead to the reduced risk of various diseases, including Alzheimer's disease, which is a neurodegenerative disease. Currently, there is no cure for Alzheimer's disease that is why there is even greater importance and need to prevent it from occurring in the first place.

— REDUCED RISK OF CANCER

In medical terms, cancer is defined as the uncontrolled and abnormal growth of cells which then spread to other parts of the body. Intensive animal research has shown that intermittent fasting can help with reducing the risk of cancerous cells and more recently; fasting has proven to have the same effect on humans as well.

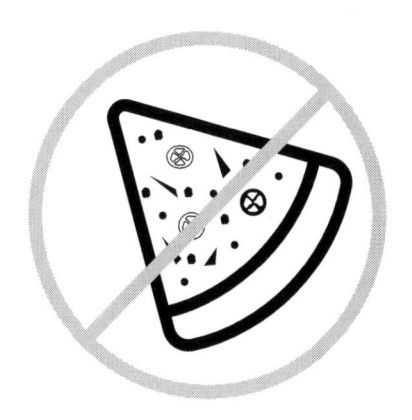

Sacrifices That Comes with Intermittent Fasting

Deciding to eat at scheduled periods could take a toll on the body. It feels like a break-down process for build-up results. This isn't an easy process, especially when it's the first time. There will be a strain and it will take the body a bit of time to adapt to it. A body that isn't trained to expect food only at certain periods in time will fight the process, but that shouldn't stop you.

Just like any other exercise or workout, intermittent fasting is going to take some getting used to. Have you ever made a meal in the kitchen and it almost seems like you have to go extremely close to the food before you can smell its aroma hit your nose, yet someone in the living room keeps telling you how wonderful your food smells?

INTERMITTENT FASTING

The reason for this is not that you can't smell the food, but it's because you've experienced this aroma for such an extended period of time, and your olfactory senses have gotten so used to it, hence it seems almost normal. Intermittent fasting is sort of the same way.

At first, there is hunger. That is always the first step, the need to eat something. This is the most common hurdle and even though it's the first, a lot of people give in. Just the thought that you would have to wait before you could eat again can initiate and promote the feeling of hunger. We are programmed to want what we can't readily have, therefore this is normal. Your body begins to crave the meals that it has been promised and when it doesn't get them, the feeding center acts to cause an increase in appetite.

This large increase in appetite starts to put your mind in overdrive. Your goal at that time is to find food to eat, and if that doesn't happen, fatigue comes in. This tiredness is normal when your body is denied food. You can think about this as a learning stage, like the training wheels your body puts on to adapt to this new system.

In essence, though, the most important question is this; is intermittent fasting worth the sacrifices? The answer; irrevocably yes! These caveats are temporary compared to the many advantages and benefits that come with it in the long run.

There are ways to prepare yourself to reduce some of the effects. It is always helpful to have a distraction which could range from a TV show to yoga and even meditation. These things help your mind focus on something other than the need to eat. After a while this regulates and the new eating and fasting pattern becomes the standard for you.

Intermittent Fasting Vs Conventional Fasting

For the earlier part of this book, we talked in detail about fasting and its history. We also discussed how influential it was in the past, spanning and surviving through the rise and fall of many civilizations and empires. We also explained that the process of fasting has been fine-tuned through the years, with new methods and ways to implement it coming up more often.

Now, in our present day, the most widely accepted method of doing this is intermittent fasting, but why is that? What has made intermittent fasting more widespread and acceptable in the present day than other types of fasting practices that have existed for millennia? This is what we'll be discussing next.

INTERMITTENT FASTING

— ABSENCE OF RELIGIOUS INFLUENCE

Fasting is commonly associated with religion. An example is in Christianity, where Christians fast during the lent period. This is a common theme in most religions as well. Fasting is also a large part of Buddhism. Here Buddhist monks learn to go for extended periods without food. This helps them veer off the path of world belongings, attachments and distractions and move towards the eternal Bliss of enlightenment that is Nirvana.

In Islam, during the holy month of Ramadan, Muslims fast as well, abstaining from food for 30 days, from dawn to dusk. These sorts of fasting also appear in a myriad of various other religions, and if you are a religious person yourself, then it is more than likely that you have participated in at least one of these fasts before.

There is nothing wrong with fasting for religious reasons, it is even encouraged, but the issue with this is that it makes something as beneficial as fasting to end up being confined within the walls of this particular religion. Therefore, for people who aren't particularly religious, therein lays the problem. They cannot readily, or may not want to join in these rituals to undergo a fast.

The concept of intermittent fasting was made devoid of religious beliefs, and therefore, since it is a neutral thing, it can be done by anyone who wants to do it. It does not clash with religious beliefs or practices and neither does it conflict with the absence of these beliefs and practices. It is a harmless exercise that brings fruitful results for all that are willing to partake in it.

— NO-DIET RESTRICTIONS

Imagine being at home in the comfort of your living room. There's a plate on the coffee table with your favorite meal placed delicately on top of it and you look at it with all the love in the world. You reach for it, but before you take a bite, your diet app rings on your phone, to remind you of your diet. You glance at your screen and then you see the list of food that you are supposed to stay away from, and right there on that list was something you forgot; the meal in front of you and your favorite food!

That would be painful for anyone and that is what dieting does. This isn't to say that dieting is a bad thing, but certain things make intermittent fasting better than it, and this is because there are no dietary restrictions.

The focus of intermittent fasting is more on "when food is eaten" than on "what food is eaten." Whatever dietary additions or subtractions are done by the person who has decided to go on the fast, he/she can still appreciate and enjoy your favorite meals, just at the appropriate time.

The best part about this is that a diet can still be combined with intermittent fasting for even better results, but it is not necessary because intermittent fasting still brings very good results all on its own.

CONSISTENT TIME MANAGEMENT

A common theme with intermittent fasting is when not what and therefore time is of utmost importance because it's the very driving force behind the concept. When this type of fasting is done, there is a form of time management put in place which restricts the amount of time in a day that food should be consumed or not consumed.

These specific periods of eating and fasting are what separate intermittent fasting from most of the other forms of fasting since most of them focus more on just the absence of meals, or at least certain types of meals.

This scheduled meal eating helps in time management and it also spills into other areas and teaches those who participate how to have control of their time.

INTERMITTENT FASTING

— FAQ WITH ANSWER!

Is intermittent fasting expensive?

Intermittent fasting is one of the cheapest exercises that you can participate in. If anything, chances are that you can even save money through it. Most people are used to eating when they want and so they can spend exuberant amounts of money on the food. With proper planning added to intermittent fasting, this process is eliminated and when meals are planned long beforehand, there is money saved.

Isn't not eating food bad for me?

The short answer is, not really. Of course, you will need food at some point, but overeating is what is very bad for you. The indiscriminate consumption of calories isn't good for your body and its immune system. By overeating, you end up giving your body too much work to do during digestion, and it isn't built for that. This is why athletes consume a lot of food, they do the work that it takes to burn it out and instead of it being turned into fat that just ends up being stored and deposited to other parts of their body, it is converted to the much-needed energy and also transformed to help muscle tissues as they are constantly worn and in need of repair.

Any normal person needs a form of activity to help with this conversion as well, and since not all of us can go through the same amount of rigorous training that athletes find themselves going through, intermittent fasting is a much better way to do this. Eating little, or at the appropriate time, combined with fasting periods that allow your body to handle cell repair and hormone regulation is the best way for your body to regulate and heal itself. It is the best way to let the physician within as it works its magic.

Dieting, in this case, would only help with a specific problem, and most times it would come with a condition that would also have to be addressed later, maybe by another diet.

What happens to our blood sugar if we decide to fast?

It is understandable to worry that the level of blood sugar in your blood will dip too low, especially when there is no food to use to replenish it. However, it is important to note that when you abstain from food, your blood sugar doesn't deplete, instead the body starts to create glucose itself. On extended periods of fasting, the body is forced to increase the number of ketone bodies it produces since the brain needs a lot of glucose to function per day. These ketone bodies act as a healthy substitute for glucose, providing the fuel that your body needs to function.

It is also important to note that since there are also periods of eating during the process of intermittent fasting; your body rarely gets into this stage. This is just to combat the common misconception that says that you will pass out if you decide to try intermittent fasting.

INTERMITTENT FASTING

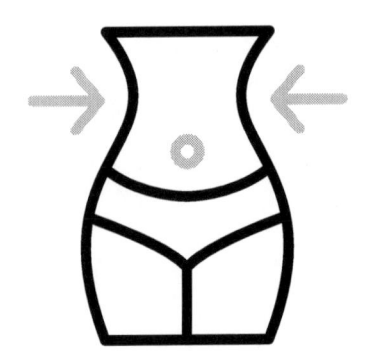

Your Weight-loss Journey with Intermittent Fasting

Susan, a 42-year-old single mother of three had to work for 40 hours a week. Added to these rigid work hours was her motherly instinct that made her want to be the one who took care of her kids, so she hired no nannies. She would come to pick her two younger kids, Billy who was only 6, and Jake who was 10. Alex, her eldest son was 13 and he came home from school by himself, but he was still too young to take care of his siblings, so Sarah did all the work.

She would put in many hours during the day and by the time she got home, she had little to no time to herself because her kids too needed her attention. She would help them with their homework, feed them and stay up with them until bedtime. Then she would catch the last hour of her favorite TV show before falling asleep, sometimes on the couch because she just didn't have the energy to climb up the stairs to her bedroom.

Her alarm would wake her up early the next morning, and she would rush to prepare breakfast for her kids and get them ready for school, while she hurried around the house getting her things so she wouldn't be late for work. She would put in her hours and repeat the entire process all over again on weekdays, leaving only the weekends as her days of rest.

Sarah was happy to do this because , she loved her kids and she loved taking care of them. She never complained about how much work it was that she had to do, as long as she could keep her family happy, she would try everything possible. The only problem was that her eating habits were all over the place because she never planned her meals according to how her day would go. She would often skip breakfast in the mornings and find something to eat at work. In most cases, this was any junk food that she could get from the vending machine in her office.

The only time that she would eat an actual meal was when she was back at home, trying to prepare dinner for herself and her family. For dinner, Sarah would often overcompensate for all the meals that she had missed. She would make a huge dinner, and eat very big portions until she was too full to move, and then, after tucking her kids in for the night, only then would she settle on the couch for some alone time. However, because of her big meal, she could never stay up too long and she would often find herself waking up in her living room the day after.

With this continuous process though, the inevitable happened which was that Sarah began to gain weight. Now, it's very normal for anyone to gain weight, it doesn't take a lot for this to happen, but with her cycle of living, this only helped to fuel her weight gain. It didn't take long for her BMI to reach the dangerous areas of the overweight category while rising steadily. She needed an immediate solution!

INTERMITTENT FASTING

A lot of coworkers told her to do the first thing that came into their minds, which was exercise. They suggested that she join a gym, which seemed like a very useless option for them to suggest since she worked in the same office that they did, and they didn't have the time to join gym either.

After going through a myriad of diets, with nothing working in the long term, Sarah was just on the cusp of giving up completely. This was until a friend of hers suggested that she tries intermittent fasting.

The moment she heard fasting; Sarah shut down the idea. She was not about to give up food just because she had gained a few pounds. It was only when the concept of intermittent fasting was explained to her that finally began to see the benefits that this idea could yield for her. For someone like her who didn't have a lot of free time to go out and join a gym, intermittent fasting became a life saver. It wasn't intrusive in her daily life and it didn't disrupt any of the things that she had to do.

All she had to do was schedule the hours of the day that she would eat, and the hours that she would fast. She did this diligently and adhered strictly to the plan. In only a short couple of weeks, just shy of a month of intermittent fasting, Sarah began to see and feel changes in her body and mind.

She didn't feel as bloated as she did before. She didn't feel hungry so often or tired as she used to earlier on. Her meals became regularized and the urge to fall asleep after dinner didn't come anymore. She felt more energetic and most importantly, her weight had drastically reduced. This was not starvation; she didn't feel hungry or sick, rather she felt healthy, for the first time in a long time.

Sarah is one of the many that can attest to the benefits of intermittent fasting. Why her story is important is because a lot of people get the feeling that they are just too busy with life to lose weight which is completely not true. Yes, they might be too busy to exercise but meal restriction and planning is a lot more

INTERMITTENT FASTING

susceptible to control. It fits in with whatever sort of lifestyle there is currently, and if that lifestyle can be altered, that's fine, but it's always nice to have this choice.

With a wide variety of intermittent fasting options available to you, whether you are too busy for physical exercises or not, intermittent fasting can play a key role in your weight loss journey.

INTERMITTENT FASTING

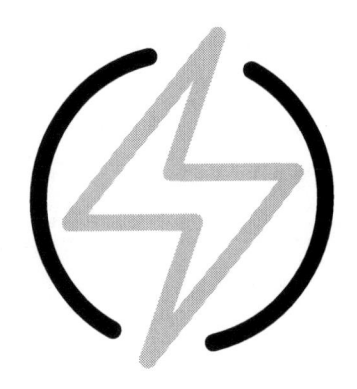

The First Changes You Notice

Everyone is looking for the results, and fast results for that matter! It's normal to go on a 30-day exercise and feel like nothing has changed, especially when you keep looking at your reflection in the mirror every two hours. It's the reason why people do a few squats and start to look at their butts in the mirror to see if there is any change. It's just liked the saying "Things only move when you aren't looking at them."

Now, how will you know if you are making any progress? How do you see these results? Well, that's easy. You just have to look out for certain things that will show that you're practicing intermittent fasting the right way and help you know that you're on the right track.

FEELING OF LIGHTNESS

One of the first things that almost anyone who has been on this journey will tell you is that they start to feel a sense of ease. You still weigh a lot at the beginning of your journey, but you start to feel a lot lighter before your scales show you the same results. This is because your body generally gets used to working, so you don't feel as heavy and bloated as you used before you started.

ENERGY INCREASE

The feeling of being light comes packaged with energy. You will start to notice that you have a lot more strength and energy to do tasks, even if they are tasks that you do on a daily basis. The earlier signs of fatigue which might be normal with people who are fasting for the first time start to fade and the improved movement of hormones and their circulation through your body starts to give signs of vitality. That is why when you talk to people who have tried intermittent fasting, they don't complain about laziness or tiredness. Instead, the common comment is about how they feel like they have been rejuvenated.

SHEDDING WEIGHT

Of course, you will lose weight, that's the point of this exercise and when you start to see the results that you had hoped for, there is a tendency to slow down and take a more laid-back approach. This can instantly put you back on the road to reverting your progress and make you lose all the wonderful changes that you have already undergone. So, when you get to this stage, and you begin to see the pounds coming off, take this as an opportunity to grind even further.

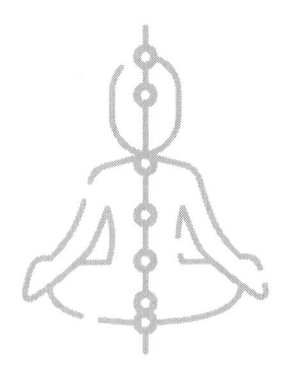

The Body Balance

Don't skip leg day! Anyone who had been in a gym had heard that saying. You don't even need a regular visit to the gym to hear it. It's a term used for people who have decided to train only one aspect of themselves, thereby neglecting several other key factors that are of major importance.

The thing is that a lot of people don't go into fasting with a complete mindset, and while this may not impede the results per se, it definitely will not help them either. What I want for you is the totality of the package. We are always trying to get better, and so it only makes sense for me to offer the best to you.

Intermittent fasting will go a long way in helping you to curb unhealthy lifestyles, but you also have to set your mind to it as well. If you are willing, and you have the right mindset, your body will respond faster, and it will move closer towards the results that you hope to get quickly.

INTERMITTENT FASTING

The ways to help this process along are simple and you should not look at intermittent fasting as an all-in-one thing. Now you might be wondering how to not do this, after seeing all the benefits it offers. One of the most common problem I've seen many encounter is when they think that the best things are the ones that can be done once and for all and this is not the case.

I think that the best things in life are the habits and beliefs that lead you to more. Intermittent fasting gives you a regulation that should spill into other habits in your life and you should take the opportunity you get to work on those things.

If it's possible, try yoga, especially when you have free time. Think of other exercises to add, to create healthier lifestyle. Your focus should not be on losing weight alone. Being healthy should be the prime goal, and nothing gets you closer to that goal than a healthy mind to work along with your willing body.

This is why finding a balance is essential to any sort of goal that has been set. Do this and there is every assurance that your weight loss journey will be a huge success.

PREPARE FOR THE STRAIN!

Ah, yes! The first few hours of fasting and you find yourself thinking about food. You never did think about it before, at least not like this. You end up questioning the entirety of the exercise that you have decided to embark on. You fight through it and move away from your kitchen, you stay away from the nearest fridge and then you try to find a distraction, something that could easily take your mind off food. It isn't easy, is it?

I think most people are still not aware, or rather do not believe that intermittent fasting can take a toll on you in the long run. Sure, there are easier ways, and people might not even adhere strictly to it, but this is not the way to go.

INTERMITTENT FASTING

I think one of the most important steps to take in intermittent fasting is preparation. This will not be all roses and daisies. It is incredibly hard to break a habit. Your body will fight back against any break in its chain of normal functioning. This is why I have hammered down on the fact that staying consistent with intermittent fasting once you have started is key. But what if you haven't? How do you break your body out of the circle that it's in and get it introduced to something new? You prepare!

Preparation could very well be one of the most important steps in intermittent fasting. It is a simple step that most people overlook. They just wake up one day and say that they are going to not eat anything till dinner time. Yet, before it is even noon, they find themselves wondering what their next meal will be. In the end, they can't make it that far and they end up breaking their fast before it even begins.

> ## How do you combat this?

The answer is this; you need to know what you are up against. You know yourself to an extent. To a few of us, it might be easy to fast for 16 hours, to others, they might not be able to go for 3 hours without food. Our body tricks us into a lot of things. That is why we eat a lot when we are bored, because eating is a regular thing, and so when you have nothing to do, your mind pushes you to what it is used to. That's why you find yourself looking through the glass door of your fridge, and wondering what snack you can take, even when you aren't hungry.

You need to be prepared for the toll that intermittent fasting will take on you. The benefits will come up, that's a given, but it comes in steps and you cannot skip steps to get to weight loss.

INTERMITTENT FASTING

Your body will try to fight back, because it is not used to going without food, so you have to be prepared to counter this. You could do this by maybe pacing yourself when you eat on the days leading up to your fast. You could time your meals, even before starting intermittent fasting completely. You could push your meals a little later than normal to see if you can get an idea of how you react to being without food.

That way when you start intermittent fasting and the strain begins to appear, you already have an idea of how long you can go against it and also how to survive it!

OVERCOMING YOUR INSECURITY

Unlike what people might say and think, no one is born with excellent amounts of confidence. That is why there are books on this subject. It is important to have a good view of the kind of person that you are. It is important to see yourself in a more positive light. We all agree to this, but how can this be done?

In this book, I won't be talking about all the things that you've probably seen on the TV or in magazine articles. I'm not trying to sell you anything so there is no reason to lie. Instead, I will outline a 3 step simple method that can help you become more confident and help you grow out of your insecurities.

Step 1 – WILLINGNESS

Your ability to want to do something is invaluable. A lot of people achieve extraordinary feats by simply putting their minds to it. Now, I'm not going to tell you something as cliché as *believing in yourself* is a fix for self-confidence issues. It might help to do so, but for now, we will start small.

INTERMITTENT FASTING

I am important. I matter and I will succeed. We do not give ourselves enough words that affirm what we want to believe. People are more likely to hammer on the things that they think they can't do than to try their luck out with the things that they can. The first step for you to get that self-confidence you need is to be willing to get it. You need to start telling yourself that you can do it, more often than not. This isn't going to magically fix you overnight, or make you forget your insecurities, but this step is incredibly important.

The reason for this is that the more you think about certain things, the more you believe them. Therefore, when you begin to put in these nuggets of positivity into yourself, you are more prone to conquering your fears and insecurities.

Step 2 – EFFORT

So, you've decided to try intermittent fasting. It never helps to do anything halfheartedly. If you do this, you counter the entire process and this can stunt your goal. The application of your entire focus or putting all of your efforts into this exercise will not automatically cancel out your insecurities. Do not be worried though, because here is how it works.

The more effort you put into something, the more your resolve grows. The more resolve you have, the more determined you are to see it through till the end. One of the greatest hurdles is not believing you can achieve the goals you have set for yourself. If you can follow the steps above, it doesn't destroy your insecurities, but it helps you put yourself forward despite them, leading you to the third and final step.

Step 3 — ACCEPTANCE

This is the final step and it is the step that requires the least from you. Your intermittent fasting journey has led you through the first two steps and now you have begun to both look and feel healthier. This step comes last because it completes the whole process.

Right now, you are going to need to accept the way you are and the fact that you've done something incredible. You committed to a program and you have succeeded. Now that you're seeing the results, your acceptance is a pat on the back, telling yourself that you've done a good job. Acknowledging that you have done well will not only increase your confidence and help curb your insecurities, it will also push you to try for more and more in your life.

The reason why these steps are important, especially with intermittent fasting is because intermittent fasting is focuses on your health and vitality. A healthy and vital mindset will help you balance this and drastically improve your weight loss game.

Make sure that you keep these steps in mind and practice whichever fits you at this moment. Self-confidence isn't built in a day. There are days when doubt will try to creep in, and you might feel like what you're doing is not working, or it might not be enough. Do not fear because your effort will pay off and you are more than enough!

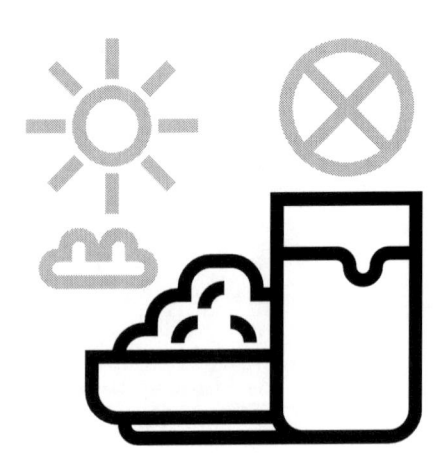

More facts about Intermittent Fasting

Added to what we have already discussed, there are still some more facts that you should know about intermittent fasting, before deciding to embark on this journey, or picking out a technique that would be best for your weight loss journey.

These are very important to know facts, at least before any decision is made. The extra information can prove to even be a motivator, and answer common questions, while simultaneously clearing up the air about several misconceptions.

THE GREAT IDEA OF STARTING YOUR DAY WITH WATER

Water, as you will see later on in this book, can be part of your fast. Depending on what type of fast you decide to do, this could be an option or a part of it.

Now that we have established that the addition of water to your fast is relative, we can continue. If you are taking water during intermittent fasting, it is a great idea to start your day with it. It is a lot healthier than most other low-calorie meals and confections that can be taken during a fast, like coffee or tea.

This isn't to dispute the importance of other confections, but the most important of them all should be water. The health benefits are tremendous and added to them, water can help you manage and, to a lesser extent, curb your hunger. Experts say that it is possible to mistake hunger for thirst, so it is best not to shy away from water.

Therefore, keep yourself fully hydrated, and start your day with a glass of water to get you on the go. Once you do this over and over, it will help you regulate your hunger patterns, and you could use this to fit into your feeding and fasting schedule.

TIPS FOR BETTER DIGESTION

One of the first and common things that may happen to you when you have decided to start your intermittent fasting journey is feeling bloated. This is often caused by focusing more on the feeding part than the fasting. Usually, this is because we feel like if we can eat enough food during our time for feeding, then maybe our hunger would not be that bad.

This fear is understandable and if you have this fear, I'm here to let you know that it's perfectly fine. It's best to ease into these sorts of things than to rush into them. Some things can help you such as apple cider vinegar.

INTERMITTENT FASTING

Apple cider vinegar has become a sort of staple in most homes, especially those who have an interest in weight loss. Chances are that if you pop open your fridge right now, you'll see a half-used bottle of apple cider vinegar just sitting there. This is because of all the health benefits it gives and one of the benefits being easier digestion.

A study conducted proved that the consumption of small amounts of apple cider vinegar at least 20 minutes before meals could help in making digestion easier. This, in turn, helps prevent or get rid of the bloated feeling.

— **SNACKS AFTER YOUR MEALS AREN'T NECESSARY**

As you will see in later chapters, there is a time to feast and a time to fast. You have the option to choose how these times are planned and the duration for each. Something else that happens a lot for most people who start fasting newly is that they tend to abuse the feeding period. Instead of the normal meals that are supposed to be taken, these meals for followed by a myriad of snacks, most of which are unhealthy.

Eating snacks during your period of feeding isn't a taboo, but it is unnecessary in most cases. This is because most of the time, they end up just being unhealthy additions that counter what you're trying to do. The feeling of hunger is inevitable, but there are ways to have a satisfying dinner that reduce this feeling a bit. This option is a lot healthier than deciding to fill up with snacks just five minutes before the end of your period for feeding.

The substitute you need is a well-balanced meal that is both healthy and able to sustain you at the same time. This is the way to do it and lucky for you, there will be a bunch of healthy, well-balanced meals that you can try out. If you can successfully stick to these added tips, your weight loss journey is sure to come to a quicker conclusion.

INTERMITTENT FASTING

FAQS WITH ANSWER!

When do I start to lose weight?

This is dependent on the type of intermittent fasting you do. Some types lead to quicker results than others and some take a while to get going. These types are picked based on individual preference and therefore they do not lead to the same types of results for everyone across the board. The types of intermittent fasting will be explained more in later chapters, along with their benefits and detailed results.

Won't starving myself help me lose weight?

Yes, it will. Technically starvation would help you shed weight, but what next? What is the point of weigh-in less if you aren't healthy?

As said before, a very big and key difference between starvation and intermittent fasting is that intermittent fasting helps you get healthy. Starvation is accompanied by extreme fatigue, nausea, depleted blood sugar levels and could even lead to brain damage due to the total absence of glucose.

On the other hand, intermittent fasting even helps to combat these effects, making it the inevitable weight loss option out of the two.

CHAPTER - 03

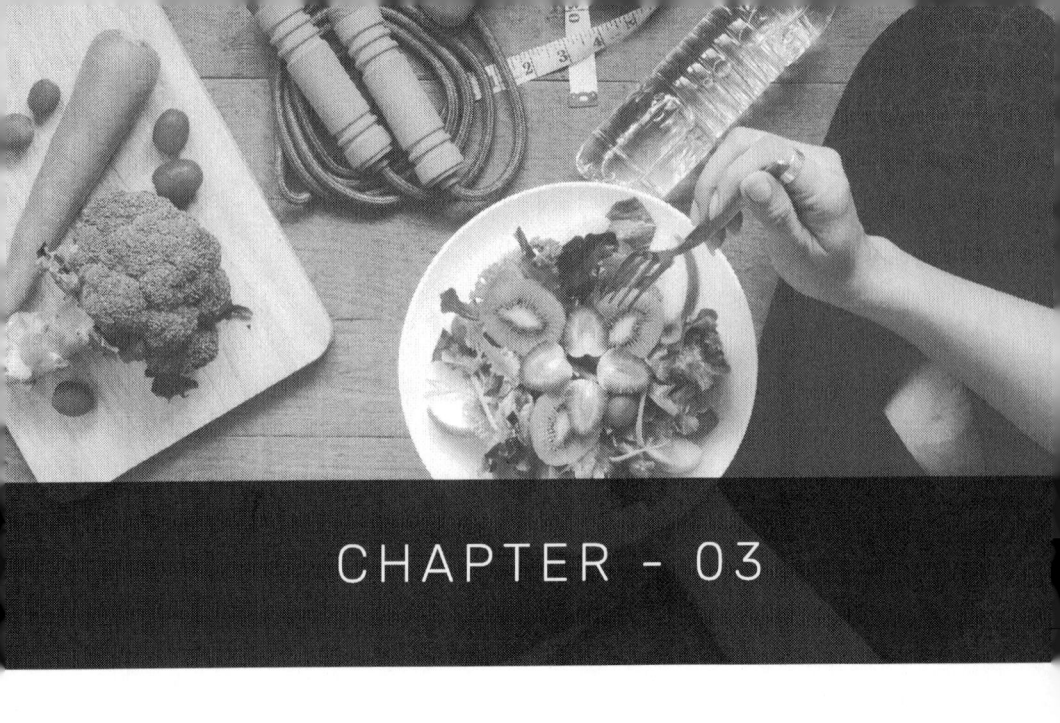

The health benefits of Intermittent Fasting

Intermittent fasting is aimed at creating a healthier person all around. This means a healthy mind, devoid of bad thoughts or worries. This healthy mind and mindset will accompany the body on its journey to weight loss, healthy living and vitality.

It is a well-recommended exercise that has consistently yielded great results in all areas of health and because of this, the benefits that intermittent fasting provides to general health has been studied intensively. A lot of resources have been put into finding out the best ways to maximize the health gains that can be gotten, and that is why intermittent fasting has been and will still be one of the most popular and important forms of fasting for a long time to come.

INTERMITTENT FASTING

This chapter will focus on two major things that involve human health, which is the heath of the body and mind. This is because intermittent fasting covers both bases accurately and that it is revered and recommended.

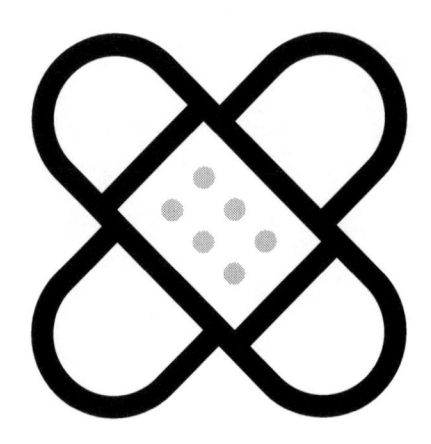

The Healing Power of Fasting In The Mind & Body

Fasting, when practiced the right way, diligently and consistently, has a lot of advantages on the entire body, mind and soul. Its healing properties are especially worthy of note as various people have reported accounts of positive changes experienced in their lives after a period of consistent fasting.

As earlier mentioned, it is important to note that starvation is different from fasting. Going too long without eating might encourage your body to begin storing more fat than necessary in unwanted places to combat the effects of starvation which would end up being counterproductive.

INTERMITTENT FASTING

HEALTH BENEFITS OF FASTING

Fasting done correctly has almost magical healing effects on the body and mind. The list of advantages is inexhaustible; however, here are a few observable changes you are sure to experience if you practice intermittent fasting consistently and diligently.

Improved Mental Capacity:

Fasting helps to clear toxins from your blood and lymph nodes which makes it easier for your blood to flow properly, untainted, to your brain and by extension, makes it easier for you to think properly because your brain can use more energy which would ordinarily have been directed to digesting food.

You might not notice this effect until after the first few days after you begin fasting. At first, you might experience headaches and slight pain because of your body trying to adjust itself but after your bloodstream has been cleared of unnecessary toxins, your brain has access to cleaner blood and you will be able to think clearer, and have more productive thoughts.

Increased Willpower:

The decision to fast requires a lot of mental strength that includes the ability to stay away from immediate gratification and focus on long-term objectives. Fasting takes a lot of patience, hard work, and commitment along with the willingness to exhibit the level of self-control required to achieve your aims.

Training Your Mind:

Sticking to your goal gives you the ability to remain dedicated to life's other challenges. You become more determined and gain the ability to remain focused on your goals, not to mention the enormous sense of accomplishment and gratification you derive from completing a task you once considered to be daunting. Your mind becomes free of negative thoughts that would ordinarily discourage you from going for the things you desire.

Rejuvenation:

Fasting takes your body through a much-needed rejuvenation process. Diseased cells are destroyed and replaced with healthy tissue. Nutrients are also noticeably redistributed all around the body as the body hangs onto precious vitamins and minerals and disposes of toxins and unnecessary materials.

Oftentimes, our body stores elements that it does not need. These elements can become excessive and prevent your organs and tissues from getting the nutrients they require to keep functioning properly. Proper fasting helps your body identify the nutrients it requires and distribute them to spots where they are needed. This process ensures that your body system remains in top-notch condition and can carry out its duties properly.

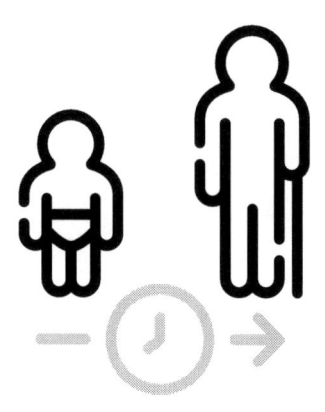

Fasting and Anti-aging

In addition to its weight loss benefits and healing properties, intermittent fasting also has amazing anti-aging effects. Fasting triggers reactions in your body that reduce the rate of aging by keeping your DNA and cells healthy by reducing cellular damage because damaged cells and inflamed cells are a major cause of chronic diseases and aging accelerates when DNA begins to wear down.

Fasting also greatly increases antioxidant levels which can help to prevent your body's cells from being broken down through reactions with free radicals. Free radicals are the unstable molecules that can damage cells therefore causing aging and other illnesses. The inflammation that comes with advancement in age is also reduced through fasting.

INTERMITTENT FASTING

— **ANTI-AGING EFFECTS OF FASTING**

When you practice intermittent fasting, it is to be expected that you will be more conscious of your calorie intake. Limiting the level of your calorie consumption reduces the risks of fatal diseases like heart diseases, diabetes, and cancer. Restricting your calorie intake also enhances energy production. All of these have a direct effect on your cells by restricting the rate of cellular damage. Your DNA isn't left out as reduced calorie intake helps to maintain healthy DNA.

It is worthy of note that conscious intermittent fasting has amazing effects on your skin. In the long run, no matter how many expensive skin treatments you go for or use, there is no denying the fact that there is nothing quite like natural healthy skin. Natural, healthy skin gives you a fresh, youthful glow.

The skin is affected greatly by the kinds of food we consume and as it is the largest, most obvious organ in the body, we need to be extra careful about the kinds of things we put into our bodies. Healthy skin is usually an indication of the state of our inner body. Glowing skin is almost always a sign of stellar health conditions.

When fasting, our body starves for a longer period than it is used to which leads to changes in metabolism. Normally, the body relies on the food we eat for energy and when it is deprived of that, it is forced to rely on other sources and through a process called gluconeogenesis, our body is forced to gain energy from stored fats and other non-carbohydrate sources like amino acids.

Fasting also causes increased levels of purines and pyrimidines in the body which then leads to higher levels of antioxidants and improves your overall body and skin health. The increase in the level of antioxidants reduces the process of skin aging.

Regulating your blood sugar, which is necessary when fasting, is also important for your skin. Collagen is the protein in our body that gives our skin its fresh appearance and although it needs sugar to function, excessive sugar causes tissues to stiffen and makes skin age faster.

Fasting also decreases skin inflammation and regulates your body's circadian rhythms to regulate the effects of inflammation more efficiently and reduce the risk of skin issues like acne and eczema.

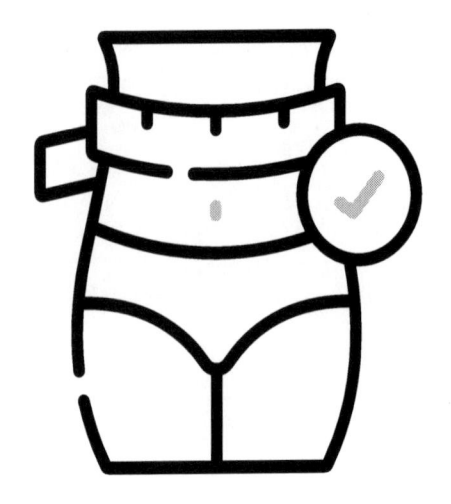

Does Your Body Detox When You Fast?

Our body is a self-healing, self-repairing organism that has various mechanisms for getting rid of toxins. Despite this, it sometimes requires an extra push to carry out its function properly. It goes without saying that both during and after fasting, certain things should be avoided to prevent their adverse effects on your body. Certain foods increase the levels of toxins in the body and damage our organs. Fasting helps to ensure that the levels of these toxins are kept to the barest minimum and eventually become non-existent.

INTERMITTENT FASTING

Some of these things that should be regulated during fasting include:

Salt:

When fasting, we are forced to limit the amount of food we consume. By extension, our salt intake is also reduced. Excessive salt in the body leads to increased blood pressure which forces the heart to work harder and increases the risk of coming down with diseases like hypertension and high blood pressure which could eventually cause heart attack. Reduced salt levels also help to reduce stress on your kidneys and prevent them from breaking down.

Sugar:

During fasting, it is advisable to stay away from high-sugar foods and sugary drinks. Excessive sugar increases your body's calorie levels. Foods that have high sugar levels give the body a quick energy boost because the sugar is absorbed into the bloodstream very fast. However, after the initial sugar rush, the sugar levels fall and you begin to feel slow and tired. Excessive sugar also makes your body retain unwanted calories. Excessive fats in the bloodstream affect your organs and clog your blood vessels, greatly increasing the risk of coronary diseases. Cutting back on sugar is an efficient way of cutting back your toxin levels.

Alcohol:

It goes without saying that alcohol should be avoided during intermittent fasting. Excessive alcohol intake is very bad for your liver and wears it out faster because it is forced to work double-time to break down the alcohol in your body. Your kidneys are also forced to throw out more fluids and vital nutrients because alcohol is a diuretic. To function properly, your body needs these fluids and nutrients. This fluid loss is what makes you feel dehydrated the morning after.

INTERMITTENT FASTING

Alcohol makes it more difficult for your kidneys to tell the difference between which nutrients are good for your body and which are toxic. Therefore, it is recommended you reduce or completely eliminate alcohol consumption during fasting.

Eggs And Meats:

These are not to be avoided completely because even though they provide much-needed proteins for some people, some find it difficult to digest them. Processed meat products are high in saturated fats and contain additives that make your body system and its organs work harder unnecessarily. These additives could increase toxin levels in the body. It would do your body good to cut back on your egg and meat intake during intermittent fasting.

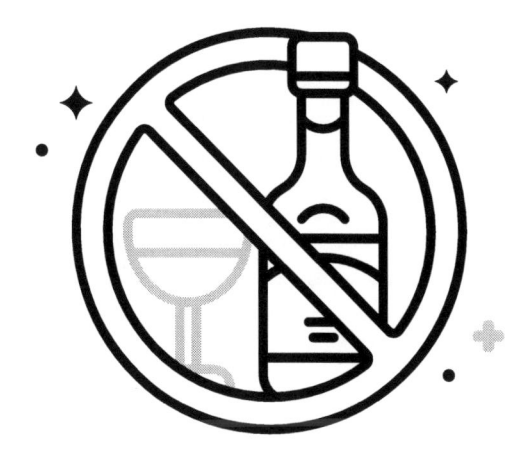

Fasting & Fighting: The Battle with Addiction

Whether your addictions are mental or physical, fasting is a good way to help you break the cycle of addiction and set you on a completely different path. Addiction is an illness or condition where we are unable to control our impulses and desire for certain substances actions, or media and the wrong kind of addiction can be dangerous to the body and mind. Examples of negative addiction are:

- Addiction to unhealthy foods, illegal drugs, or alcohol.
- Addiction to sex related content
- Addiction to technology and media such as phones, gaming, or television.

INTERMITTENT FASTING

Most people might not view some of these addictions as negative but they become dangerous when they start to have adverse effects on your productivity and the overall quality of your life. Say, for example, a person has alcohol addiction, they might be able to control it in the beginning but it might get to a stage where the signs become more obvious and affect the person's ability to function efficiently, particularly in cases where the person develops a reliance on alcohol to perform daily tasks. Addiction is a serious problem and should be treated as one. However, the first step is to recognize that one has an addiction that needs to be dealt with.

Addiction can also cause serious illnesses to a person. Drug addiction can lead to mental impairment and reduced cognitive function and Certain drugs like cocaine have been known to affect sleep cycles. Addiction to junk food can lead to excessive consumption of toxins and unnecessary calorie build-up in the body which have direct effects on the body organs and also wears them out easily. Addiction to devices can make it difficult to focus on tasks and important things in life. Fasting is a great way to break habits that may not be considered beneficial. The period during which one undertakes a fasting regime can serve as the much-needed push to identify areas where change is required alongside the kind of changes needed and the factors to put in place to ensure that these changes are carried out.

Fasting has been proven to be the most efficient and sophisticated willpower workout available. Breaking addictions requires a lot of mental strength. Intermittent fasting requires willpower to build and strengthen the level of your patience and ability to focus on a goal. By becoming good at fasting, you develop self-control and you will be able to control other aspects of your life, particularly your addiction. No matter how deeply embedded, practicing consistent fasting will make it easier for you to overcome any addiction. Fasting has also been proven to greatly dissipate the craving for alcohol, nicotine, caffeine and other addictive drugs.

INTERMITTENT FASTING

The process is easier if you set rewards and goals for yourself for every set period when you can resist your craving for your addiction. When you reward yourself, your body and mind become more willing to do the work to resist your addiction.

FAQS WITH ANSWER!

Does intermittent fasting really help with weight loss?

Although more research is needed to determine whether intermittent fasting leads to real, sustainable weight loss, the 2018 study published in Nutrition and Healthy Aging postulates that alternate-day fasting produces better weight loss effects than time-restricted fasting even though time-restricted fasting is easier to stick to than alternate-day fasting. Current data suggest that intermittent fasting can lead to 5 to 9.9 percent body weight loss. The meaning of this is that intermittent fasting coupled with exercise is a good place to start if you intend to start your weight loss journey.

Does intermittent fasting slow aging?

In 2014, Cell published a study that suggests that intermittent fasting and calorie restriction slows aging. When you make a conscious effort to control the number of calories you ingest, you are also helping your body save its cells and prevent damage to your DNA. By extension, this means that your body has more energy to focus on healing damaged tissues and making new cells while strengthening or discarding worn-out ones as required.

INTERMITTENT FASTING

How does intermittent fasting improve metabolism?

Fasting and eating healthy helps your body maintain a healthy metabolic balance which boosts your body's immunity. This doesn't mean that you should practice excessive fasting as it can have negative effects on your overall health and cause more health challenges which would end up being counterproductive.

Intermittent fasting causes a hike in your body's antioxidant levels. These antioxidants have a generally good effect on your body and skin. There is no doubt that a healthy metabolic system will have a direct effect on your outward appearance.

How does fasting affect your brain and mind?

One of the more interesting effects of fasting is the results it has on the functioning of the brain. It has been stated earlier that fasting serves to cleanse your body of toxins. The absence of toxins in your blood helps your brain function properly and gives you a renewed ability to think clearer thoughts. Some studies have found that fasting helps those with Parkinson's and Alzheimer's. Fasting stimulates the production of certain proteins that are essential for learning and provide protection against the cognitive decline that comes with age.

Does intermittent fasting help the immune system?

Fasting essentially "flips a regenerative switch" that restores the immune system. Even though the body system can heal itself, there are times when we may need to help it do its job by staying away from substances that might hinder it. Through intermittent fasting,

INTERMITTENT FASTING

we become more conscious of the things we put into our bodies and the effects they have. Fasting gives our body, particularly organs like our kidneys and liver, the much-needed break it requires from dealing with an inordinate number of toxic elements daily.

CHAPTER - 04

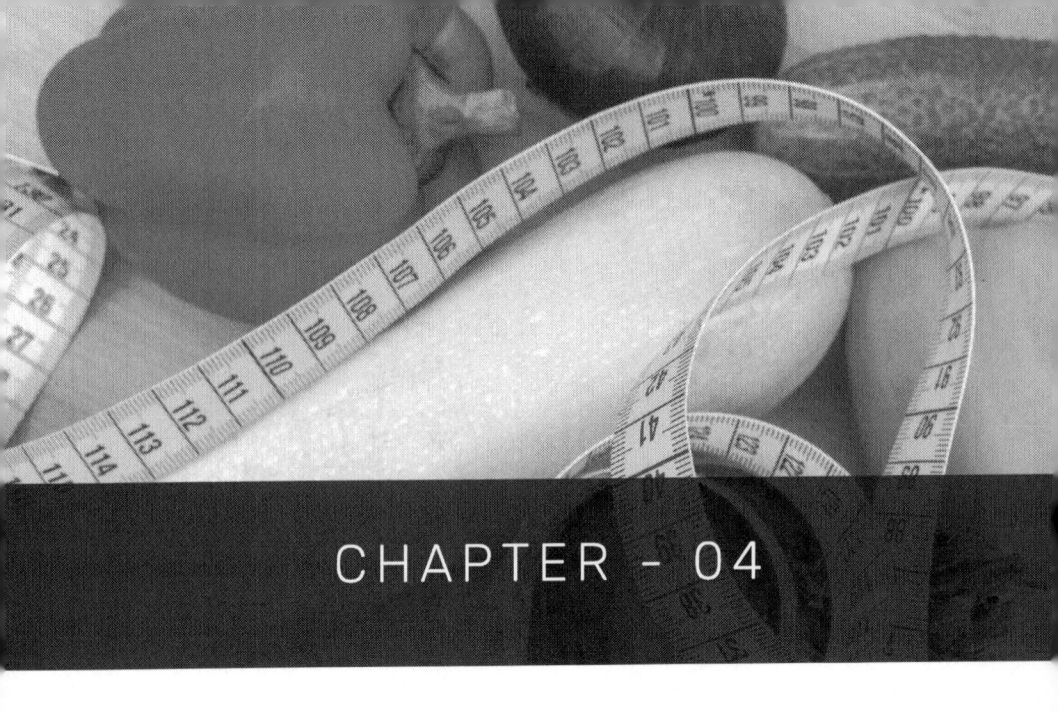

Who can practice Intermittent Fasting?

Ultimately, anyone can fast and there is no specific right way to practice intermittent fasting. Any decent fasting regimen will require a large amount of discipline and paying careful attention to nutritional requirements to get results you can be proud of.

Some people may find intermittent fasting too daunting or demanding. Some may find themselves unable to stick to its requirements. There are also those for whom the risks of intermittent fasting outweigh the benefits by far due to their health conditions. For some, it could be dangerous.

INTERMITTENT FASTING

The category of people for whom intermittent fasting is safe include:

- People who have practiced "dieting" before. This refers to people who have prior experience with monitoring their food and calorie intake.
- People who are single or do not have children.
- People whose jobs will permit them to have a low performance while they adapt to a new fasting regimen.
- People who are actively trying to lose weight are also allowed to practice intermittent fasting provided they do not do it excessively and are sure they have no underlying conditions which might make it difficult for them to stick to their fasting plan. For these people, fasting is best practiced alongside physical exercise. For optimum results, working out should occur towards the end of the fasting window, just before the time allotted for eating arrives.

There is a category of people who can practice intermittent fasting while exhibiting a bit of caution. These are:

- People who have children and/or are married.
- People who compete in sports or athletics.
- People who have goal-oriented or performance-oriented jobs.

These sets of people are subject to conditions that make it much harder for them to stick to fasting protocols than most people. Intermittent fasting could mess with their ability to achieve their set goals and mess with their overall performance output. Sudden intermittent fasting isn't advisable for all women as it has been known to cause anxiety, sleepless nights, and irregular periods due to disruption of hormonal balances.

INTERMITTENT FASTING

People who should not practice intermittent fasting at all are:

- Pregnant women.
- People with a history of eating disorders.
- People who are chronically stressed.
- People who do not sleep well/insomniacs.
- People who are new to diet and exercise.
- Persons below 18 years of age .
- People who have been diagnosed with chronic health conditions.
- People with severe anemia.

Pregnant women have high energy requirements and are not advised to practice intermittent fasting as this kind of deprivation is not healthy for both mother and child. Unlike normal people, pregnant women are technically eating for two. Staying away from food for extended periods deprives their body of the much-needed nutrients required to sustain the mother and unborn fetus. When the fetus does not get as many nutrients as it needs, it could lead to severe congenital health conditions and defects.

People who have a history of eating disorders like anorexia and bulimia are advised to stay away from intermittent fasting of any kind because practicing fasting could lead them back down the rabbit hole of intentional starvation. Even though they may start fasting with good intentions, there is still a high possibility that intermittent fasting could trigger their eating disorders all over again.

People who are under severe stress or are not sleeping are also not advised to practice intermittent fasting as their bodies require nurturing and more energy. Fasting under these conditions is not favorable because it leads to more stress.

INTERMITTENT FASTING

People who are new to dieting and exercise are advised to take it easy when practicing intermittent fasting. Some fasting regimens are stricter than others and it is not healthy for a person who isn't used to dieting to immediately start with the stricter methods of fasting.

Youths under the age of 18 are another group of people who are not advised to try intermittent fasting because they are prone to take the process to extreme levels which would ultimately be dangerous to their health or result in eating disorders.

People who have been diagnosed with chronic health conditions like diabetes or hypertension need a well-focused, therapeutic technique to manage their conditions. Since their bodies aren't at their optimum levels, they might be unable to access extra energy sources as required.

People who are suffering from severe anemia are not advised to practice intermittent fasting as it could worsen their condition. Anemia is a medical condition in which the ability of the cells to transport oxygen is greatly reduced. People with anemia need more energy than normal people because their cells are weaker. Practicing fasting can lead to increased weakness, faintness, shortness of breath, and sometimes death if care is not taken.

If you think you would like to fast anyway, it is recommended you consult your doctor before starting and if your doctor advises you not to proceed with the fasting, it is best you adhere. Similarly, people who work in shifts might find it difficult to adjust to their fasting plan or balance their feeding and fasting windows.

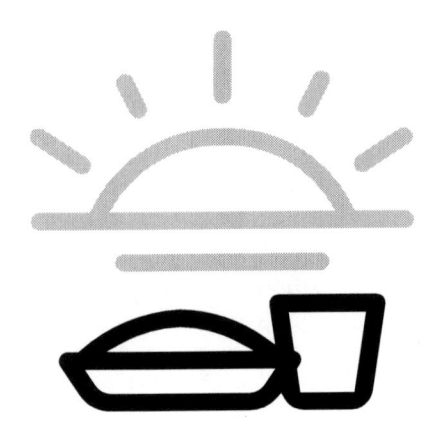

Why Should You Practice Intermittent Fasting?

As discussed earlier, intermittent fasting has numerous advantages which cannot be overlooked. Even though fasting is still a somewhat controversial topic in the medical field, many recent studies prove that fasting can and has offered a lot of potential health benefits.

For example, besides helping to boost the immune system, fasting helps to slow down the growth of cancerous cells. These cells thrive better when they have access to sugar and certain other elements. Fasting denies them access to these minerals and reduces the rate of cell multiplication and proliferation. An experiment carried out on mice and published in Science Translational Medicine showed that five out of eight cancer types in mice responded to fasting alone without the introduction of chemotherapy. The combination of fasting with chemotherapy produced much stronger effects on cancer than the use of chemo alone.

INTERMITTENT FASTING

FAQS WITH ANSWER!

How does intermittent fasting work?

For some people, intermittent fasting works best when they stop eating at a particular time during the day and completely avoid eating at night. Certain studies have proven that the body is likely to store more fat when you eat indiscriminately and excessively at night. Although the time of eating may differ from person to person, many people have reported success when they restrict their eating times to between 10 am and 6 pm. It is advised to try to avoid eating after 6 pm.

Are there beverages that can be consumed during the fasting period?

Yes, you are advised to drink plenty of water during the fasting period when you are not eating solid food. Water helps you to conserve energy and it also helps your metabolic processes. It also helps to maintain homeostatic balance in your body. Soups like vegetables, chicken or bone broth can also be taken. Soda and beverages with high sugar content or caffeine should be avoided. Taking beverages that are high in sugar would be counterproductive to the fasting process and may carry risks. Coffee and tea can be consumed as long as you do not add sugar to them.

INTERMITTENT FASTING

Is it good to exercise while fasting?

According to Harvard Health, exercising while your body is in a fasted state helps to burn fat. The body requires a source of energy to function while exercising. Usually, the body's energy comes from sugar molecules that are stored as glycogen molecules in the liver. The absence of this source forces the body to take its energy from other sources such as fat stores in the body. This is even more reason why you should exercise close to the end of your allotted fasting time as the body's cells are more deprived of energy at that point.

Can people who are taking medication fast?

No. It is not advisable for people who are taking medication to try fasting. Fasting while taking medication might tempt you to skip a dose during your fasting period which might worsen your health condition and cause complications. Not to mention the fact that while taking medication, your body's cells would require more energy to act alongside the chemical components of your medication to fight diseases. Fasting makes it more difficult for your body to access the nutrients it needs to work with the components of your dose.

Is intermittent fasting a must for everybody?

No. It isn't compulsory for everyone to practice intermittent fasting. We all have different systems that respond differently to different regimens. It is one of the many lifestyle changes that can improve your health.

Should kids fast?

It is not advisable to let kids fast as they do not yet have the discipline to know when to stop. You would also be exposing them to the risk of eating disorders and ulcers. Children need a balanced diet to grow properly and letting them skip meals is not advisable.

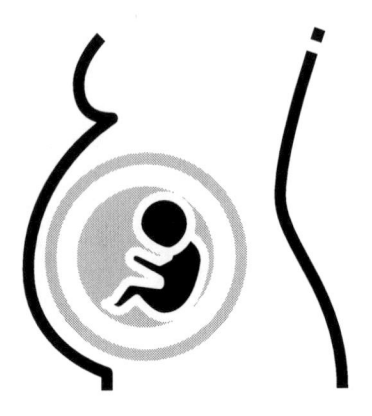

6 Reasons Intermittent Fasting Is Not for You

As crazy as it may seem there are certain restrictions when it comes to intermittent fasting, these restrictions aren't because of race or tradition or even religion. There are also not because of dietary constraints like lactose intolerance. No, those don't affect intermittent fasting exercises. The restrictions I'm talking about are, more than often, health restrictions.

Some medical conditions require that you eat. There are also other things you need to do that require you have food in your stomach. These things are what we are about to look into.

IN THE CASE OF A PREGNANCY

Fasting should not be done when you are pregnant. The adjustments that your body has to make during the period of intermittent fasting might not always be the best to handle when pregnant. The strain might prove to be too much, leading to unwanted complications. The same goes for whether you're trying to get pregnant. This is safer though, but you should make sure that there is no chance that you are already pregnant before you start intermittent fasting. If you have already given birth and you are breastfeeding, it is advisable to halt all attempts at intermittent fasting as well.

PRESENCE OF AN EATING-DISORDER

An eating disorder is a condition that should be looked into before you embark on intermittent fasting. If you have had any instances of an eating disorder in the past, chances are that it might come again when you start to restrict your meal times and start staying without food for extended amounts of time. That is why it is not advisable to start intermittent fasting when this condition is or could be present.

UNDERWEIGHT CATEGORY

People who possess a Body Mass Index (BMI) of below 18.5 fit into the underweight category. It is not advisable to start intermittent fasting when you are already below the recommended normal weight range. The extra weight loss might be too much for your body to handle and you end up becoming sick and fragile, bordering on anorexia in worse cases. This can lead to serious health issues, so if you belong to this category, intermittent fasting would only be an option when it is added to an aggressive weight gain diet, targeted specifically at you. Here, intermittent fasting ceases to be a measure for weight loss, rather it just becomes a health care regimen.

INTERMITTENT FASTING

— IMMUNE SYSTEM ISSUES

A compromised immune system will not be able to handle the toll that fasting takes on the body. It is best to consult a healthcare professional, or a personal doctor on how to proceed if this is an issue, to avoid complications that could end up leading to very serious issues.

— LONG TERM MEDICAL CONDITIONS

Persistent conditions and long-term health issues such as anemia, diabetes, cancer and epilepsy should be taken into account if a fast is to be considered. Intermittent fasting in this case should only be done if there is express permission from a doctor, and should never be done without proper supervision. If there isn't even one of these, the health complications are too great of a risk to take.

— SPECIFIC MEDICATION

There are specific medications that you can be on that require a healthy and more than moderate amount of food for the strain that it takes on your body. Blood pressure medication is just one among these, and so fasting is not recommended for people in this situation.

INTERMITTENT FASTING

FAQS WITH ANSWER!

Should I continue my fast even when I fall sick?

This depends on what sickness it is. Some signs come with intermittent fasting that isn't symptoms of a sickness. Like the fatigue, or the dizziness that comes initially as you try to adapt. These are very routine and they pass eventually as you start to get used to the exercise.

However, if you already have a pre-existing medical condition, it is best to have that treated first before starting the fast. Intermittent fasting might not act as a cure, but it acts as prevention. So, there is a higher chance of not getting that sickness again if you embark on intermittent fasting.

Still, if your medical condition cannot be cured, then it would be best to refer to what has been said above and consult your doctor to know if intermittent fasting is a viable option. If not, then it would be best to seek other means of help.

Can I continue my fast, even after taking medication?

This depends heavily on the medication which is ingested. I mentioned earlier that some medications require a lot of nutrients to work, and so they need a lot of food to do their job. If there is an absence of this, the drugs take too much of a strain on an already fragile body, and because of that, a fasting technique will not be enough to provide the extra nutrients that are needed.

INTERMITTENT FASTING

If your medication is somehow light, maybe for a small headache or something similar, then fasting could continue, but if the medication is more than that, then it is important to consult a health care personnel before even thinking about intermittent fasting.

What benefits does exercise have when added to fasting?

Anyone who has this in mind is already aiming for the optimum results. Exercise on its own is a great way to lose weight. The wide varieties of exercises that exist only help to widen the range of people who can do them. As explained earlier though, there isn't always time. People's busy schedules usually end up conflicting with this and that is why intermittent fasting comes more recommended.

Although, a combination of these two could only serve to help, it is almost a surety that your desired results will come even faster. However, you should pace yourself.. Intermittent fasting will also put enough strain on you, any physical exercise that is too strenuous will wear you out and make you require food and that will immediately end your fast.

The Possible Health Risks

There are two sides to a coin and there is always a fifty percent chance that a flipped coin will land on either side. This means that a bet made on one side has just a halfway chance of winning and that is how most things are in life. There are two sides to most things, some good, some bad, but like the coin, it isn't always as clear-cut. Sometimes the bad things outweigh the good, and sometimes it's the other way around. Intermittent fasting is an example of the latter.

There are always risks in every endeavor, but the question remains. Do the benefits outweigh the risks?

In intermittent fasting, the correct answer is YES. The benefits outweigh the rails involved by far, but that doesn't mean that there aren't any. It is a good thing to know what you're getting yourself into, and because of that, the possible risks are things that you should be aware of before making your decision to start intermittent fasting. The most common ones will be outlined and explained below.

MOOD CHANGES

This is quite common and although it is downplayed as not being a serious issue, it should be taken into utmost consideration. Most of the mood swings that occur during intermittent fasting are a result of your body trying to balance and regulate your hormones. In this process, your mood gets affected and you start to feel irritated and sometimes even sad, with no control over it whatsoever. Another thing that can lead to these changes in your emotional state is the lack of food. Hypoglycemia or low blood sugar can occur during periods of fasting. This in turn makes you irritable as well.

A study in 2016 was conducted on 52 women who went on intermittent fasting. It showed that these women were more easily annoyed during their 18-hour fasting period, than their period of non-fasting. Even though they got annoyed and we're easily irritable, the study reported that these women attested to better self-control, sense of self-worth and pride when they had accomplished their task.

HEADACHES

Headaches and feelings of light-headedness are common side effects that accompany the first few days of the fasting exercise. Researchers have shown though, that these headaches usually occur in the frontal area of the brain. The pain is also usually moderate or mild in intensity.

Another way these headaches can come easily is if the individual has such a medical history. Therefore, if you are susceptible to headaches, chances are that when you start intermittent fasting, you are going to encounter these headaches. Thankfully, this only lasts for a while before the body learns to adapt and then the headaches disappear.

MALNUTRITION

Intermittent fasting in itself does not cause malnutrition, however, if it is done incorrectly, intermittent fasting just ends up becoming starvation, and that in turn causes malnutrition.

Another thing is neglecting the feeding part of the exercise. Feeding part is important as the fasting part and if there is a recommended number of calories to be consumed, these calories should not be skipped or run away from.

If you deliberately restrict calories to the extreme in an attempt to get your results even quicker than before, then malnutrition can set in and this will lead to health complications in the space of a very short time. To fix this, or even avoid it, you will need a carefully drawn-out intermittent fasting plan that you will strictly adhere to. The help of a health care professional also comes highly recommended.

SLEEP DEPRAVITY

Some studies show that altered sleeping patterns may arise during fasting. Disturbances in sleep such as not being able to fall asleep or not being able to sleep for long periods are common side effects of intermittent fasting.

A study conducted in 2020 observed 1,422 people that took part in intermittent fasting that lasted within the range of 4 to 21 days. At the end of the study, the research showed that about 15% of all who participated showed signs of sleep-related issues due to fasting. This was reported more than the other effects that fasting could lead to

INTERMITTENT FASTING

— FATIGUE

This has been talked about before, but the reason it keeps coming up is that the misconception that people have when this is said is just regular tiredness. Fatigue however is more than that. In severe cases, people could pass out because of their exhaustion, or start to display reduced cognitive functions. It is also a gateway to things like migraines, nausea and even vomiting.

It is good to note that extreme fatigue occurs mostly in cases where intermittent fasting isn't done correctly. When the proper guidelines aren't followed, this could cause fatigue and in order to prevent this, a lot of preparation should be put into the process of intermittent fasting. You should know yourself and your limits as well. They are important to understand the threshold of things that you can do. This way you do not end up overexerting yourself and wearing yourself out.

Part

03

When to Eat

CHAPTER - 05

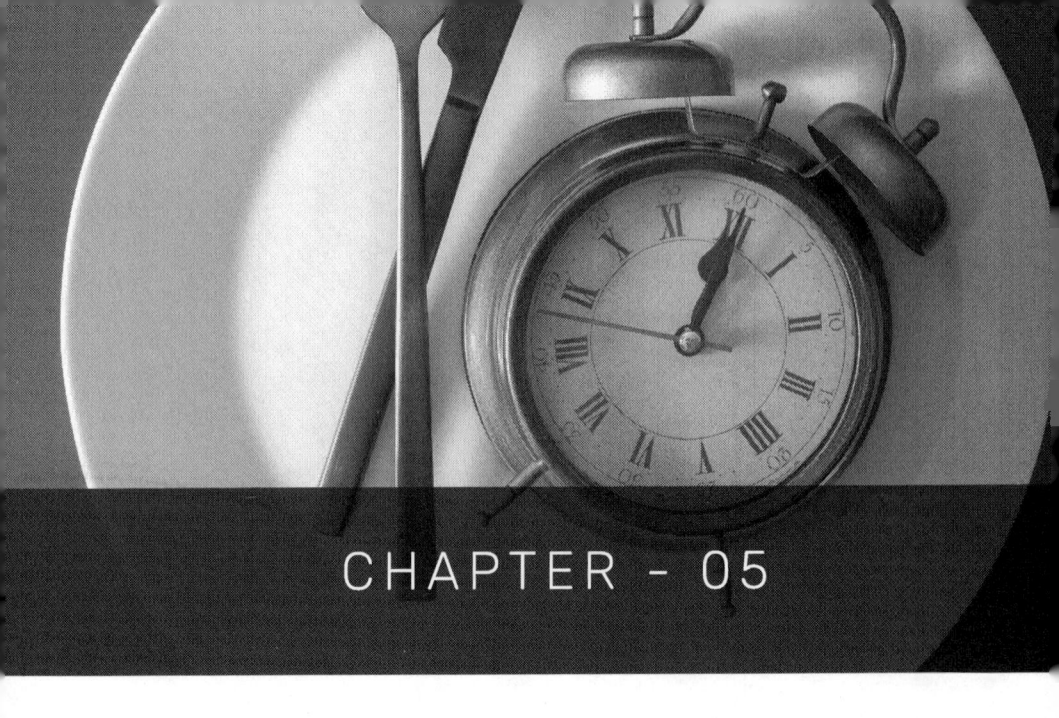

When should you eat?

Julie, a 46-year-old real estate salesperson in San Francisco was one of the most sought after in her field. She had a way of closing every deal, no matter how impossible it looked. The word around her firm was that she could sell anything to anyone and a matter of fact she did! She always tried to look at the part, and act the part as well. Julie was tough as nails, having grown up as the oldest sister of four younger brothers.

She was a business mogul with little time for anything else. She wasn't overweight, she perfectly fits into the normal weight category and she knew this, so it didn't occur to her that she had any heart issues. This is until one day when she fainted just as she was about to leave the house to work. Her neighbors caught sight of this and rushed her to the hospital and the diagnosis was that she had high blood pressure caused by elevated stress levels.

INTERMITTENT FASTING

The truth was that people saw her for what she presented; a calm and confident working woman who could tackle anything, but the fact was that there was stress lying just beneath the surface. She had too much work to do and while she enjoyed this, it still took its toll on her.

Now, this was a wake-up call for her and she knew that she needed something that would help control her stress levels. Meditation and yoga weren't in the cards for her because she did not have that sort of free time that would allow for regular intervals of exercise. This was the point where the concept of fasting began to appeal to her. It was something she could do while on the go. She wouldn't have to take time off from the job that she loved and she would also be able to work well enough to get the promotion that she was gunning for.

What did Julie do? Julie decided that she was going to do a 24 hour fast and she accomplished it. She didn't feel any changes though, at least not in her health. All she started to experience were migraines and dizziness. She read that these were just normal symptoms of a fast and that her body would get used to it eventually, so she tried again after a few more days. She went on another 24-hour fast and waited to see if she would get any results. There wasn't a lot of difference in her weight though, but that wasn't what she was doing this fasting exercise for.

Julie, being as ever-persistent as she was, tried again, and still, there was nothing. Just more signs of fatigue, nausea, and now her sleep was heavenly being affected. She could no longer get a good night's sleep or be able to sleep for extended periods.

In all, she started to feel a lot worse than she had felt when she started and her stress was going through the roof. She decided to quit fasting altogether. She told her friend about it and her friend laughed at her efforts, clearly seeing the mistake that she had made.

INTERMITTENT FASTING

Most people are like Sarah. They hear about the benefits of fasting, read about it a bit without truly understanding the concept of fasting, and without any consideration for their bodies, they jump right into it, expecting a miracle of some sort to happen. That's not how this works though.

You need introspection. If Julie had studied herself well enough, she would have known that if she wanted to fast, her focus should not be ongoing without eating, instead, it should be on when to eat.

By now intermittent fasting, or at least the basics of it, is not a new subject. You should already have an idea of what it is and how it works. This part of the book is more focused on the implementation of intermittent fasting. Here you will find out the numerous ways to do it and from them, you can pick which one would work best for you.

At this point, you know that intermittent fasting deals more with the question of when rather than the question of what and that is what this part I'd dedicated to. We will find out when to eat and when to fast, by going through the various methods and meal plans to find out what would be more convenient for you to do.

This begs the question, when do you eat? Intermittent fasting has two parts. It has the fasting period and the eating period. These times are alternated between each other. The times allocated to each part are decided upon before the fast, with more emphasis put on the fasting period over the feeding period. The feeding periods are just as important as the fasting periods. This is what keeps the balance between both of them, knowing that they carry equal importance.

Julie's problem was not because she fasted for 24 hours straight, the issue here was fasting for so long, only to go back to her sporadic feeding habits and overconsumption of junk food. These weren't helping her, and they countered

INTERMITTENT FASTING

her periods of fasting. The pattern that would have helped her more would have been any form of intermittent fasting that focused on a certain balance each day. The one that we are about to cover now is one of such methods and it would have fit her more.

As you read through these methods of intermittent fasting, look at yourself and think about what would be best tailored to you. It is only you that can get the results you want.

Your guide to Time-Restricted Eating

Intermittent fasting is a compound term for all the fasting techniques which require alternation between periods of fasting and periods of feasting. Under this umbrella term lies various methods of fasting and each of them is similar, with a few key differences to distinguish them. However, each fasting plan under intermittent fasting has fasting hours that are more compared to the usual fast that happens overnight. The first of these that we will be covering is called **time-restricted eating.**

Time-restricted eating, just like the name, means restricting the amount of time that meals can be consumed. An example of time-restricted eating is when you decide to eat for only an 8-hour window during the day, maybe between the hours of 9:00 a.m. to 5:00 p.m., then you only have this time to eat whatever you have chosen.

INTERMITTENT FASTING

The 16 hours that are left in the day are strictly for fasting, so during the time outside of your eating window, you are not allowed to eat anything. This is then repeated every day for as long as the fast is supposed to last.

This method is highly recommended and widely used too, and it is also one of the most popular types of intermittent fasting because of how inexpensive it is to practice. It doesn't require a lot of preparation in terms of spending and as such this has to be the best step for beginners and those who are planning on easing into the intermittent fasting scene.

INTERMITTENT FASTING

Why should you practice Time Restricted Eating?

Some people eat all day, right from the time they get out of bed till the time when they go to sleep. For these kinds of people, switching to time-restricted eating could make them eat less.

There is research that supports the claims that time-restricted eating can reduce the number of calories you consume per day. Also, a particular study discovered that when some healthy adult males restricted their eating to a 10-hour window, the number of calories they consumed daily was reduced by about 20%. Further studies also showed that young males ate roughly 650 less calories per day when their food intake was limited to a 4-hour window.

Even so, some studies show that certain people do not eat fewer calories when they practice time-restricted eating because even if you are eating within a

INTERMITTENT FASTING

shorter window, you are likely to eat a normal day's worth of food if you choose to consume foods that are high in calories during your feeding period.

The implication of this is that time-restricted eating may not work for you if you are not conscious of the kinds of food you take in during your eating window.

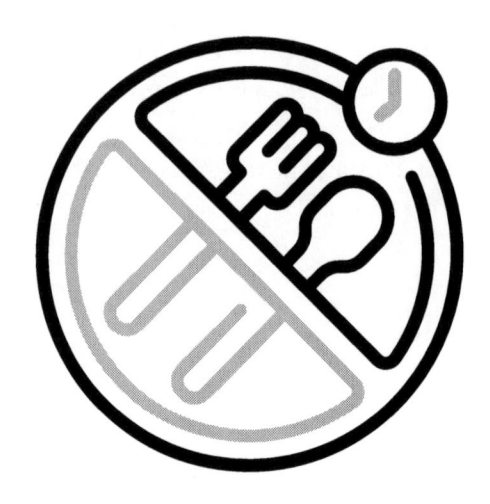

Proven benefits of Time Restricted Eating

When practiced correctly, time-restricted eating has many good implications for a person's overall well-being. Some of these are:

— WEIGHT LOSS

Studies have been carried out on both normal weight and overweight people where their eating was restricted to a 7–12-hour window. Both groups reported weight loss of up to 5% within 2-4 weeks.

Other studies, however, carried out on normal-weight individuals did not report any weight loss using similar duration of eating windows.

INTERMITTENT FASTING

Experiencing weight loss with time-restricted eating will depend on your ability to manage and monitor your calorie intake within your eating window.

If you can eat fewer calories per day while practicing this pattern of feeding, then you are likely to experience weight loss with time.

HEART HEALTH

Some substances, when present in the blood, can greatly affect the risk of you getting heart disease. One of such substances is cholesterol.

There is a substance referred to as "Bad" LDL(Low-Density Lipoprotein) cholesterol which increases your risk of heart disease while "good" HDL (High-Density Lipoprotein) cholesterol decreases your risk of heart disease.

According to a study, it was discovered that four weeks of time-restricted eating within an 8-hour window reduced "bad" LDL cholesterol by 10% in both men and women.

Still, some other research using similar eating window lengths did not report any specific differences in the cholesterol levels of their participants. The disparities in the results of both groups of normal-weight adults may have been due to differences in weight loss which may have arisen as a result of the amount and kind of calories consumed by both groups.

Those who lost considerable weight using time-restricted eating had improved cholesterol levels while those who did not lose weight did not have improved cholesterol levels.

Slightly longer eating of about 10-12 hours may also improve cholesterol levels. In cases like these, studies carried out on normal-weight people over four weeks have shown that "bad" LDL cholesterol levels were reduced by up to 10-35%.

INTERMITTENT FASTING

— BLOOD SUGAR

Your health is affected by the amount of glucose (sugar) present in your blood. It is never a good idea to have too much sugar in your blood as excessive sugar can damage some of your organs and lead to diabetes.

Some of the studies carried out on normal-weight people reported reductions in blood sugar of up to 30% but just as with cholesterol levels, this was determined by the kinds of foods that we're consumed within the eating window. Taking high sugar foods may increase rather than decrease blood sugar levels.

INTERMITTENT FASTING

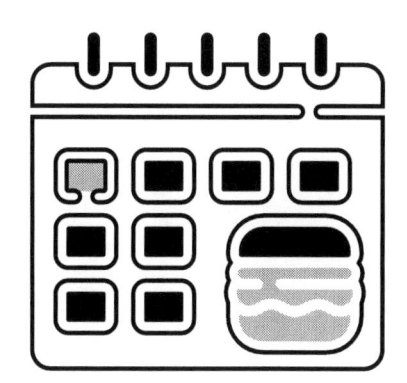

Practicing Time Restricted Eating

Time-restricted eating is one of the simplest methods of fasting. You simply need to choose a specific number of hours during per day which you can consume your food and calories. If you plan to improve your health and lose weight, the number of hours allocated to eating should be considerably less than the number of hours you'd normally allow.

What this implies is that if your normal pattern is to eat your first meal of the day at 8 a.m. and you continue eating throughout the day until 9 p.m., you eat your food within a 13-hour window every day.

For you to use time-restricted eating effectively, you will need to reduce the number of hours. You might decide to close the eating window to about 8-9 hours. By extension, you'd have to eliminate a few of the snacks or meals you normally consume. Most people use windows of 6-10 hours per day as this

INTERMITTENT FASTING

time frame is more effective than others. Shorter eating windows are generally more effective than longer eating windows.

Time-restricted eating majorly focuses on when you eat as opposed to what you eat, hence, it can be combined with any kind of diet if you wish such, as a low-carb diet or a high-protein diet.

In conclusion, as a dietary strategy that places more focus on the time you eat rather than what you eat, effective time-restricted eating would require you to limit your eating window to a shorter window during which you can eat less food and also lose weight.

The good news is that time-restricted eating has good benefits for your heart health and blood sugar levels.

CHAPTER - 06

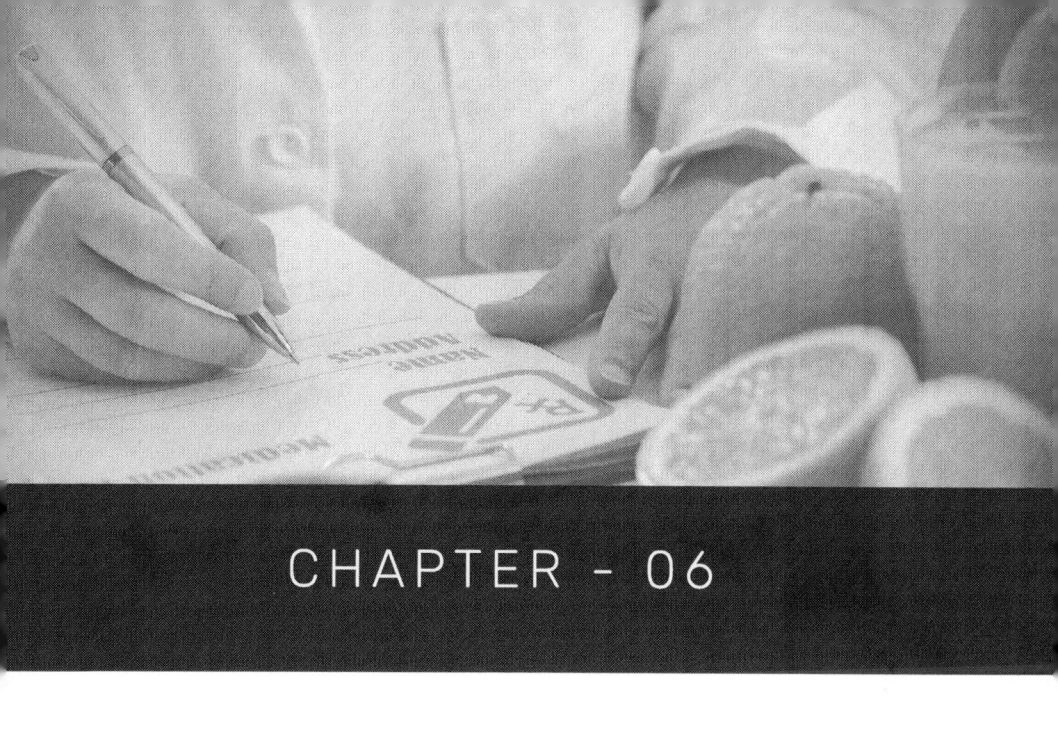

The Fast Diet - 5:2 Diet Plan

Now that you understand time-restricted fasting or time-restricted eating, the next topic that we will go to is the 5:2 diet. This is more commonly, especially in recent times and you are about to find out why that is.

INTRODUCTION TO THE 5:2 DIET

The 5:2 diet, also known as "The Fast Diet" or the "twice a week method" is at present the most popular method of intermittent fasting. It was made popular by the British journalist Michael Mosley.

INTERMITTENT FASTING

It is referred to as the 5:2 diet because out of the seven days in a week, five are normal eating days while on the other two days, calories are restricted to 500-600 per day.

This diet is often considered as a lifestyle because it carries no requirements about which foods to eat but places more focus on when you should eat and most people find it easier to stick to this diet than the usual calorie-restricted diet.

Let's Start the 5:2 Diet

The 5:2 diet is very easy to explain and practice. What this means is that 5 days a week, you can eat normally without worrying about restricting or limiting your calories.

On the remaining two days, you then reduce the number of calories you ingest to a quarter of your normal daily needs. For men, this is 600 calories and for women, this is 500 calories.

You can freely choose the two days of the week you would like to restrict your calories intake but you must have at least one normal eating day in between.

For example, a common way of planning your eating calendar weekly is to fast on Mondays and Thursdays using only two or three small meals and then eat normally for the remainder of the week.

INTERMITTENT FASTING

You must understand that "eating normally" does not translate to your binge eating or eating just anything. If you eat junk food excessively, you may end up gaining weight rather than losing weight. Eating normally means you eat the same amount of food as when you hadn't been fasting.

— USING THE 5:2 METHOD FOR WEIGHT LOSS

For those who need to lose weight, the 5:2 fasting method can be extremely effective when practiced the right way because it ensures that you consume fewer calories than you usually do.

This is even more reason why it is important to make sure that you do not try to compensate for the fasting days by eating a lot more on the non-fasting days.

Intermittent fasting, in general, does not lead to more weight loss than regular calorie restriction if you do not monitor your calorie intake closely.

Similar fasting methods close to and including the 5:2 method have shown a lot of results in weight loss studies. Recently, it was discovered that the 5:2 fasting method can lead to a weight loss of 3-8% within a 3-24-week period. Participants of the study were seen to lose 4-7% of their normal weight circumference, implying that they were able to lose harmful, stubborn belly fat. This method causes a smaller reduction in muscle mass than that usually experienced with normal calorie restriction methods.

The Exact Way of Eating on Fasting Day

There isn't an exact guidebook for what or when to eat on designated fasting days. Some people function better when they begin their day with a small breakfast while others prefer to eat as late as they can.

In general, there are two meal patterns followed by people practicing the 5:2 method:

- Three very small meals consisting of breakfast, lunch, and dinner.
- Two slightly bigger meals: only lunch and dinner.

Because calorie intake is limited to 500 calories for women and 600 calories for men, it would make more sense to correctly maximize your calorie budget wisely within limit.

INTERMITTENT FASTING

Your focus should be on nutritious, high-protein foods containing high-fiber which will make you feel full without needing to consume too many calories.

Different kinds of soups are a good choice on fast days because they make you feel fuller than foods with equal calorie content or the same ingredients when present in their original form.

Some foods that may be suitable for fast days are:

- A generous portion of vegetables.
- Natural yogurt with berries.
- Boiled or baked eggs.
- Grilled fish or lean meat.
- Cauliflower rice.
- Soups such as; miso, tomato, cauliflower or vegetable soups.
- Low-calorie cup soups.
- Black coffee.
- Tea.
- Still or sparkling water.

There is no one right way to eat on fasting days. As such, the need to experiment is paramount in order to find out what works best for you. For best weight loss results, it might be good to combine this fasting method with a little bit of exercise.

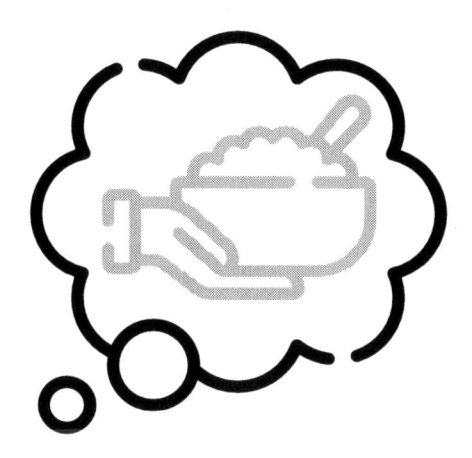

ALERT: Controlling the Overwhelming Hunger

At the initial stage of fasting, you should expect to have episodes where you feel overwhelming hunger within the first few days and you should also expect to feel weaker or slower than normal.

The good thing is, hunger tends to fade away quickly especially if you distract yourself by keeping yourself busy with work or any other activities. It is important to note that this hunger is a result of your body trying to adjust. Most people have reported that after the first few days, it becomes easier to continue with the fast.

If you are not used to fasting, it might be good for you to keep a small snack close by during your first few days of fasting if you feel faint or ill.

INTERMITTENT FASTING

If the illness doesn't subside and occurs repeatedly during those first few days, you should get something to eat and ask your doctor if it would be okay for you to continue. Please note, not everyone can cope with intermittent fasting.

In conclusion, the 5:2 method is a very easy and an effective method of losing weight, while at the same time improving your body's metabolic processes. A larger percentage of people find it easier to stick to this method than a regular calorie-restricted diet. For people looking to lose weight, the 5:2 method is a good method to try!

CHAPTER - 07

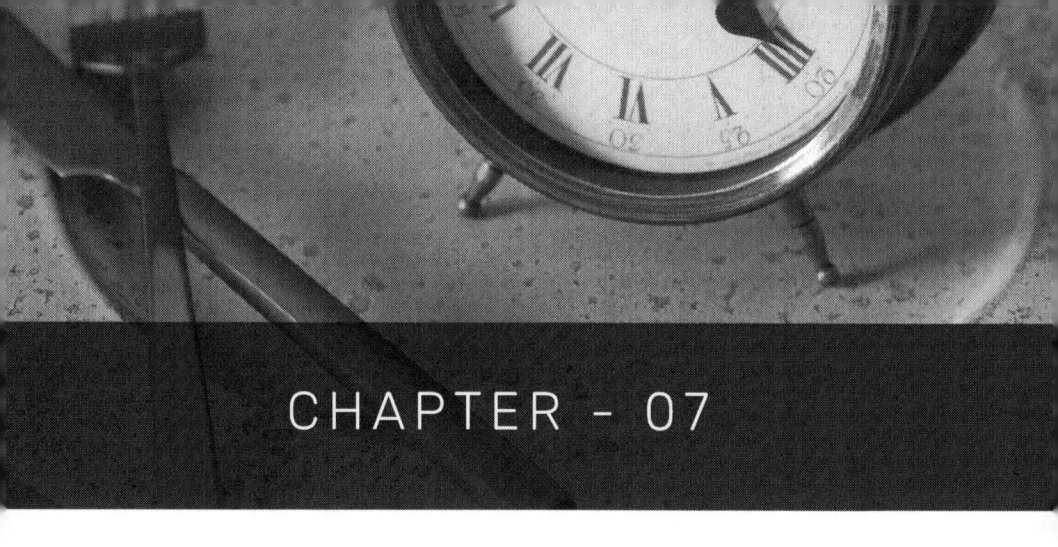

The alternate-day fasting & 24 hours fasting

DAY 1	12 AM - 7 PM	7 PM - 12 AM
	Normal Eating Schedule	Fasting

DAY 2	12 AM - 7 PM	7 PM - 12 AM
	Fasting	Normal Eating Schedule

DAY 3	Normal Eating Schedule

DAY 4	12 AM - 7 PM	7 PM - 12 AM
	Normal Eating Schedule	Fasting

DAY 5	12 AM - 7 PM	7 PM - 12 AM
	Fasting	Normal Eating Schedule

DAY 6	Normal Eating Schedule

DAY 7	12 AM - 7 PM	7 PM - 12 AM
	Normal Eating Schedule	Fasting

INTERMITTENT FASTING

Alternate day fasting (ADF) is one of the ways of practicing intermittent fasting. Using this diet, you are allowed to eat whatever you want on your non-fasting days while you fast every other day.

The most popular fasting version of this method is one where you have "modified" fasting which allows you to eat about 500 calories on your fasting days.

Alternate day fasting could help with weight loss and also help to reduce risk factors that may be related to heart disease and type 2 diabetes.

INTERMITTENT FASTING

Essentials of Alternate-Day Fasting

A DF, alternate day fasting, is one of the intermittent fasting methods. The basic approach to ADF is that you fast on one day while you eat what you want on the following day.

This means that you only have to watch what you eat half the time. On your fasting days, for example, you are allowed to drink as many calorie-free beverages as you want. Some of these beverages are:

- Water.
- Unsweetened coffee (without sugar).
- Tea.

INTERMITTENT FASTING

If you are sticking to a modified alternate-day fasting method, you are free to eat close to 500 calories on your fasting days (i.e. 20-25% of your normal energy requirements).

Popularly, the most well-known version of this diet is called "Every Other Day Diet" by Dr. Krista Vardy who is known to have carried out a large number of the studies available on alternate day fasting.

The health and weight-loss advantages of ADF are independent of whether the calories consumed on fasting days are consumed as lunch or dinner or scattered throughout the day as small meals.

Most people find it easier to stick to alternate-day fasting than other dieting types. Most of the studies carried out on alternate-day fasting used the modified version of consuming 500 calories on fasting days. This method was found to be a lot more sustainable and effective than doing dull fasts on fasting days.

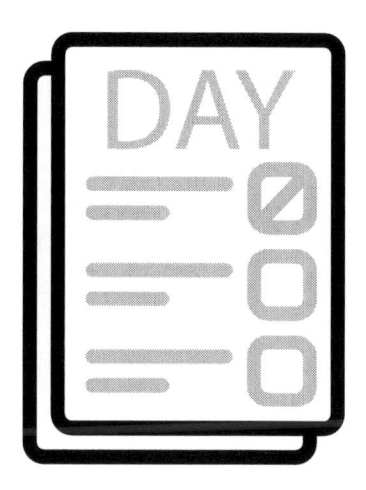

Alternate Day Fasting and Hunger

The results of studies carried out to show the effects of alternate-day fasting on hunger are slightly inconsistent. Some studies show that hunger usually goes down eventually on fasting days. However, the research generally agrees that modified alternate-day fasting using 500 calories per day is a lot more tolerable than going through full fasts on fasting days.

One of the studies that compared alternate-day fasting to calorie restriction showed that alternate-day fasting increased the levels of brain-derived neurotrophic factor (BDNF) after 24 weeks of follow-up.

INTERMITTENT FASTING

BDNF is a protein that plays a role in body weight maintenance and energy balance. Researchers have further concluded that alternate day fasting induces long-term changes in BDNG and these changes may cause improved weight loss maintenance.

Certain animal studies have shown results proving that ADF results in decreased amounts of hormones responsible for hunger along with increased amounts of hormones which bring about satiety in comparison with other diets. One other important factor to take into consideration is compensatory hunger which is commonplace with traditional calorie restriction.

Compensatory hunger is a term used to refer to increased amounts of hunger that our body goes through as a response to calorie restriction. This type of hunger makes people eat a lot more than they would usually need to, when they eventually permit themselves to eat.

Studies carried out on alternate day fasting have shown that it does not increase compensatory hunger as is the case with regular calorie-restricted diets. Most people who try modified alternate-day fasting say that they experience diminished levels of hunger after the first two weeks. Eventually, fasting becomes effortless.

■ RELATIONSHIP BETWEEN ALTERNATE DAY FASTING AND AUTOPHAGY

One of the most important effects of alternate-day fasting is that it stimulates autophagy. Autophagy is a process through which old components of cells are recycled after being degraded. This process plays a major role in keeping certain diseases at bay such as; heart diseases, cancer, infections, and neurogradation which thrive through cell multiplication.

Certain animal studies have shown over and over that both long and short-

INTERMITTENT FASTING

term fasting increases autophagy and could be linked to a reduced risk of tumor growth alongside delayed aging. In addition, fasting has been proven to increase the lifespan of rodents, yeasts, worms and flies. Furthermore, cell studies have shown how fasting increases autophagy to stimulate effects that help to ensure you remain healthy and also increase your lifespan.

All of this evidence has been supported by studies carried out on human populations which show that alternate-day fasting diets can reduce oxidative damage and increase antioxidant levels, bringing about changes that serve to increase lifespan. All of these findings need to be carefully studied to find out the best way to carry out alternate day fasting for maximum benefits.

INTERMITTENT FASTING

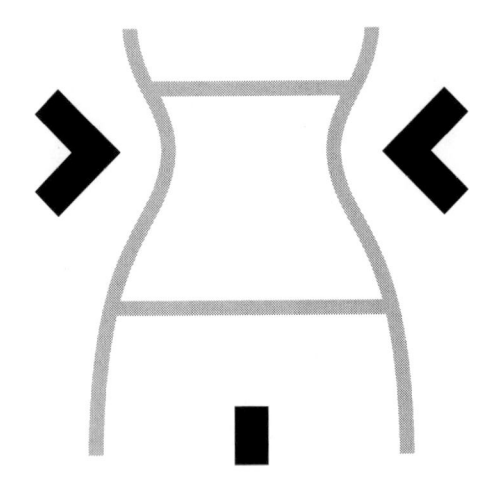

Is Alternate Day Fasting Safe for People with Normal Weight?

Alternate day fasting isn't good for weight loss alone; it can offer extensive health benefits for people who have normal weight.

Although it ultimately brings about a decrease in fat mass, alternate day fasting has been found to have a considerable effect on the metabolism and overall well-being of people who aren't suffering from obesity. It has been known to be good for heart health and cancer prevention particularly if participants carefully watch the kind of food components they consume. Not all elements are necessary; an excessive amount of some elements could result in health complications and ADF can help to manage and curb these effects.

INTERMITTENT FASTING

In conclusion, alternate day fasting is a very good way to lose weight for many people although it is not advisable for children, pregnant women, people who have a history of eating disorders, lactating people, or people who are living with rare disorders such as Gilbert Syndrome.

It does have a lot of benefits over regular calorie-restricted diets which is one of the reasons why it is very popular. It has been held responsible for many positive improvements in health. One of the best things it has in its favor is that it is very easy to stick to and be consistent with.

INTERMITTENT FASTING

What Happens in a 24 Hours Fasting?

Most people might not be interested in this particular chapter because they feel it's just too hard. However, what you need to remember is the difference between fasting and starvation. This process of 24-hour fasting has a lot of hidden parts that a lot of people are oblivious to and this is the reason why they find it particularly difficult.

The 24-hour fasting regime is longer than the other methods which we have discussed in the previous chapters. As its name states, the fasting period in this is for an entire day; the full 24 hours. This isn't for everyone though because as you know now, what matters most is finding a fasting regime that works for you.

INTERMITTENT FASTING

People who have tried the shorter intermittent fasting regimes will attest to the fact that hunger begins to increase on day 2. It is usually at this point that the hunger reaches its peak, and after that, it is easier to continue as the hunger drops gradually.

You've seen all the benefits of intermittent fasting and at this point, you begin to wonder if all of this is true. Will it work? The actual question should be; will it work for you?

Each person is different and as a result of that, their needs are different. Most people would say they want to try the intermittent fasting and they end up doing it wrong on many levels. They might not even do the proper research, unlike what you are doing right now as you are reading this book.

So, yes, there is a chance it won't work for some people. However, this is unlike the list of people who are not supposed to try it. This section of the book is based on people who might have chosen the wrong one for themselves and in these cases, there are different factors involved. The two broad categories which are always of the debate are the topics of clean fasting and dirty fasting.

This is a highly contested topic in the fasting community and on almost any forum that talks about intermittent fasting, there is a debate on clean fasting and dirty fasting. That is just how popular they are and hopefully, this part of the book will help with giving a more general idea and mindset.

CHAPTER - 08

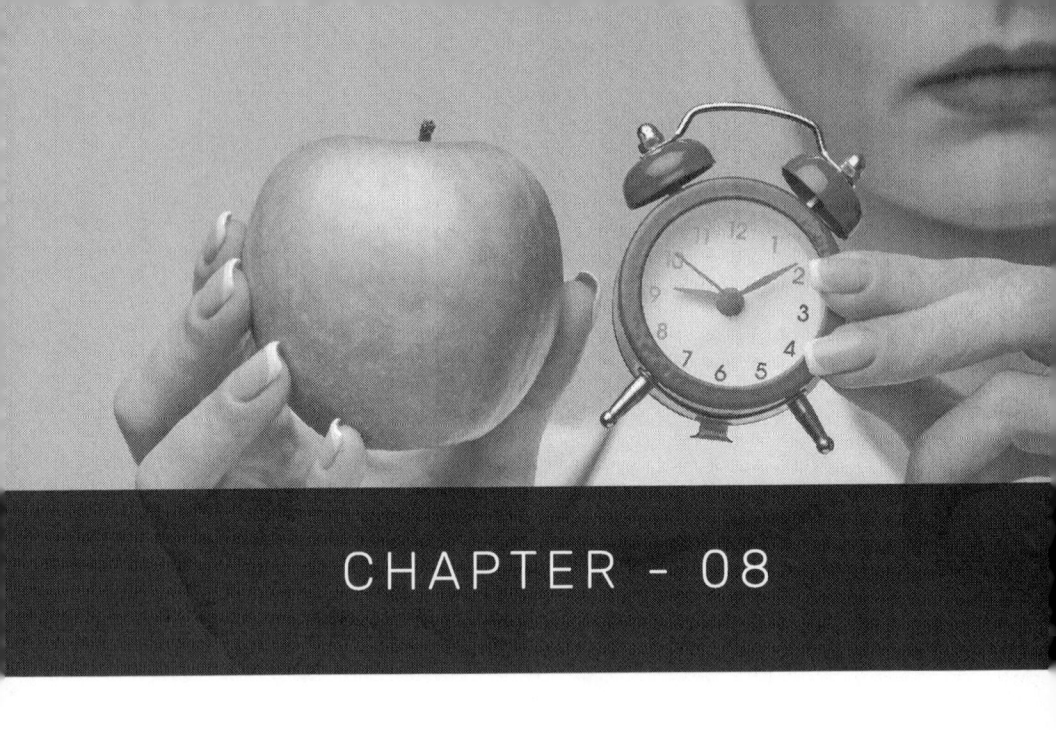

Clean Fasting Vs Dirty Fasting

aurel and Jeannie had always clashed. Most people assumed that the friends always got into their squabbles because they didn't live far enough apart from each other. They both lived just outside of each other's front door, on the same floor of their apartment building. That wasn't the only thing that these women shared though; they worked together at the same telecommunications office as call attendants, which means that they sat at their desks all day at work and they would even make a competition of this.

Both women would sit for hours and hours and try to answer and attend to as many phone calls as possible per day. They would tally up their totals at the end of each day to see who won. The loser of this bet would be the one to buy their "going home snack" as they called it, from the coffee shop very close to their apartment building.

INTERMITTENT FASTING

This was a tradition for them and something that they always looked forward to. This "going home snack" wasn't anything grand as it was usually something small like a piece of cake, or a bagel. Just something harmless that one could enjoy while the other was forced to watch and hope for a better day next time. This had become a norm for them and none of them opposed it. They were quite good at their jobs and because of that, neither one of them ever had a straight week of winning. Even if it was one day, one would always find a way to come out on top and this only fueled their drive for competition

One day, Laurel decided that she wanted to enroll in an online baking class, and a after a while Jeannie enrolled too. They were able to complete the course at the same time, and soon a new tradition began. They would tally up their calls for the week and at the very end, the person with the most calls cleared would get a bake baked for them by the other. This new tradition soon became their undoing.

The first person who had to bake a cake was Jeannie and instead of hating the fact that she had lost, Jeannie put in her efforts to make the sweetest cake possible for her best friend but to show that she was better at baking. This was a bit hard for her because Jeannie was not as good with measuring quantities as Laurel was. After a lot of hard work, she was eventually able to create a wonderful cake that even Laurel couldn't deny that it was excellent. Laurel made herself lose the following week so that she could see if she would be able to bake a better cake than Jeannie, and she actually did.

Both women mainly kept to themselves so as the cakes started to fly in, they ate them alone, and soon, after short few months, the effects began to show. Both women began to feel constipated and bloated. They felt tired just by sitting down and doing absolutely nothing. Their jobs, which had been an easy thing to do and had been one of the things that they looked forward to on working days, became a burden to them.

INTERMITTENT FASTING

They still baked, but at this point, it felt more like a chore than anything else. And maybe most noticeable of all, both women had put on considerable weight. They were hard-working people though and they decided that their new and sudden weight gain would not stop them from doing something about it. So, they went through the usual phases.

First, they went to the gym on weekends. They would push themselves each time they had to chance and soon it turned into a competition of one trying to outdo the other. This ended up costing both of them as they would get tired very quickly, without even completing a full workout. When this eventually failed, they decided to try what they thought was the next best thing. It was while they were still researching the proper diets to take, that they stumbled upon fasting.

They were instantly taken by the idea and a lot more research brought them to learn more about intermittent fasting and it seemed like the best option for them. They didn't have any long-term medical issues, and they also didn't have any signs of sicknesses from their parents or anything, so it seems like the perfect thing. Things were going great until they hit a roadblock. What type of intermittent fasting should they do?

Laurel leaned towards clean fasting. To her, it seems like what would bring her results even quicker and it felt like the only way to get the very best out of fasting.

Jeannie on the other hand felt like she was more compelled by dirty fasting. It appealed to her more that she wouldn't be going on a total fast, and still be able to get the benefits.

This was where both friends clashed and it was time for them to make a decision, which type of fasting was better. Before we get to their answer, we need better knowledge of both clean and dirty fasting.

INTERMITTENT FASTING

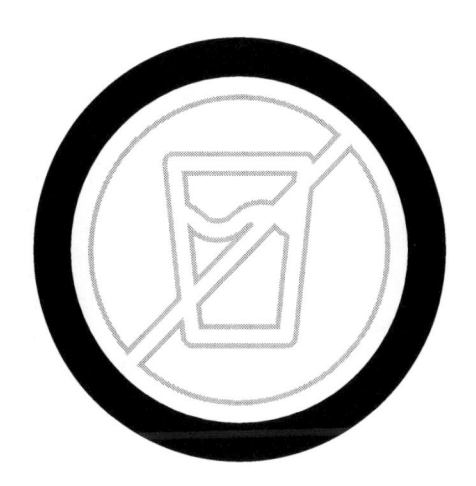

Should I choose Clean Fasting?

To understand why laurel felt like clean fasting was better, it is important we first analyze what clean fasting is since we've already covered the topics of intermittent fasting and time-restricted feeding. Clean fasting is a term used to describe time-restricted feeding where there are no calories consumed. Instead, what is consumed are calorie-free drinks and beverages.

Examples include;

- Tap water.
- Sparkling water.
- Mineral water.
- Black tea
- Black coffee

INTERMITTENT FASTING

A couple of things on the list above possess a few calories, like black tea and black coffee which have about 5g per cup, but this is completely negligible and has no effect whatsoever. The reason for this lack of calorie intake is because we are trying to prevent the triggering of an insulin response.

During clean fasting, hydration is very important, hence a person should consume a lot of water. Black tea and coffee are acceptable, but that is about it. There should be no additives, added sweeteners, or artificial enhancers of any kind. A common misconception is the addition of lemon in a clean fast or drinking lemon water. This defeats the purpose of the clean fast in the first place, as herb and fruits are not allowed in a clean fast.

The coffee that is consumed during this time should also be done in moderation, as caffeine is a natural diuretic and copious amounts trigger the creation or formation of urine. Excess caffeine could lead to excess urination, which in turn would lead to dehydration, and that is not something that should be gotten especially during a fast.

When the amount of coffee consumed is regulated, this becomes safe. So, even here pacing is key. Clean fasting gives the feeling that you're doing absolutely everything possible to stay healthy and as a result of this, people who do clean fasting feel like doing anything else would impede the progress that they have already worked to make for themselves.

That is why people like Laurel will find it hard to see any other type of fasting to be as relevant as theirs. In their eyes, what sort of fasting would be better than when you are doing absolutely everything the way it should be without trying to cut corners?

This reasoning is not necessarily wrong but the problem with this is the fact that they only see things from their point of view. That is why we will cover the point of view from the opposing team as well. What this will do is give us the much-needed insight that is required before any sort of comparison.

INTERMITTENT FASTING

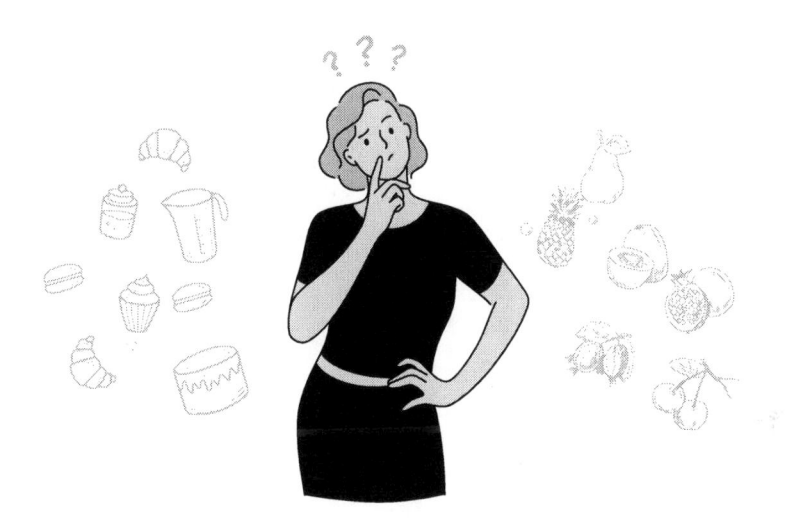

What is considered as Dirty Fasting?

Unlike what the name would suggest to most people, dirty fasting does not mean 'dirty' as in 'bad', this is a popular misnomer. It is more along the lines of a slightly different approach to intermittent fasting and time-restricted fasting.

Dirty fasting involves the consumption of a certain number of calories during your fasting period. However, this should be 50 calories because anything above that is eating. Adding a bit of sweetener to your tea or adding lemon to your water, all qualify as dirty fasting.

INTERMITTENT FASTING

Examples of things that you can eat during dirty fasting are stated below;

Ingredients	Carbs (g)	Calories (Cal)
Water with added juice of a lemon	0	14
1 cup of bone broth	3	40
Sugar-free gum	0	0
1 teaspoon of honey	6	20
1 teaspoon of MCT oil	0	38
1 tablespoon of cream	0	30
1 tablespoon of 2% cow's milk	1	18
1 tablespoon of maple syrup	14	17
1 tablespoon of aspartame	7	35
2 tablespoons of almond milk	1	10

Nothing on the list above has more than 50 calories in it, and as a result, when these are consumed, the fast isn't broken, but only regarded as dirty fasting. Clean fasting is the absence of all the above entirely. Research shows that the addition of lemon to your water or the adding of a tablespoon of honey in your tea will not remove your body from its fasted state. This means that the effects are pretty much the same, with only major difference being that you can eat and have a bit more to consume during your period of fasting which is unaffected.

Something like aspartame is an artificial sweetener. Even with this, it leaves your insulin levels unaffected, that's why your body isn't kicked out of the fasting state that it is in. It doesn't affect your insulin or blood sugar, even in diabetic patients.

However, it is important to note that these things do not add any increased advantage to your fast. There are no lasting effects that make this to be a better option than clean fasting. These additives are put in just for the added options and for taste.

INTERMITTENT FASTING

Other examples of artificial sweeteners that can be considered are Splenda and sucralose. Both of these also do not trigger insulin responses. However, this doesn't mean that they have good qualities that help health. But on the other hand, they have no diverse effects either, and so are harmless during your fast. They are just added options that a lot of people go for depending on the kind of thing they want.

This is the sort of research that Jeannie did before embarking on dirty fasting. She made sure to get all her facts right and closely measure her calorie intake so that she would not pass the limit of what she was supposed to be consuming.

INTERMITTENT FASTING

Which one is the best?

Just like the case with Laurel and Jeannie, there is a lot of debate when it comes to these two topics. Almost any forum or seminar or video that mentions these two fasting methods tends to pit them against each other. People are always trying to find out which one is the better fasting method, especially if they are already implementing one of them as their chosen method of intermittent fasting. So, it remains. What is the answer to this fasting conundrum?

To find that out, how about we look at the results of both women after they completed their first round of time-restricted fasting?

Laurel had stuck to her clean fasting diligently, except for the few non-calorie liquids that she took while on her fasting period (these were liquids that she

INTERMITTENT FASTING

would sometimes stay without) she took nothing else. She did this continually over 2 months, being consistent with the program throughout that time.

Before the end of the first month, all the uneasiness that she had felt at the start had finally subsided. She no longer experienced feelings of nausea and light-headedness when she stayed away for food for those extended periods. Her whole body started to feel lighter as well, and the bloated feeling she got whenever she went to work was gone. She made a point not to check her weight until the entire two-month period was over, but she didn't even need to get there before she knew that her new method of restricting her calories was working tremendously.

Laurel also boasted of better focus when it came to the tasks that she needed to accomplish. This made her stand even more strongly behind her verdict that clean fasting was the best method of meal restriction. She couldn't imagine how the few extra calories that Jeannie took were going to help matters. At the end of the two-month-long fasting period, Laurel had lost 12 pounds!

Jeannie had planned out everything. She didn't want to make mistakes that would cause her to lose even a day of fasting, as such, she had carefully measured out what she could add to her list of things that were okay to consume during her period of fasting.

After a few weeks, she began to get into the groove of things, and soon she had her specific rhythm. The fasting headaches and the irregular sleeping patterns had come, but the extras that she took seemed to help her body combat them, and since they were little, they didn't affect her fasting as well.

This worked well over the first month, and when Jeannie looked to her best friend, Laurel, she couldn't understand why Laurel had decided to completely lay off calories, and sometimes stay without taking anything at all. She tried to convince her to come over to the side of dirty fasting, but all her efforts fell on deaf ears. She decided that her results would prove everything to Jeannie at the end of the two months, and sure enough, she got her results.

Before that thigh, Jeannie could boast of better cognitive function. One of her issues at the beginning, which was lack of concentration, had bolstered to great heights. One of the most significant things that improved, at least in Jeannie's opinion, was her ability to measure quantities. It had been a big deal for her because of the continual need to make sure that she didn't eat more calories than she was supposed to, and the constant practice of this measuring helped her with this.

Probably most important of all was her weight. She had lost about 11 pounds after the entire period of fasting.

INTERMITTENT FASTING

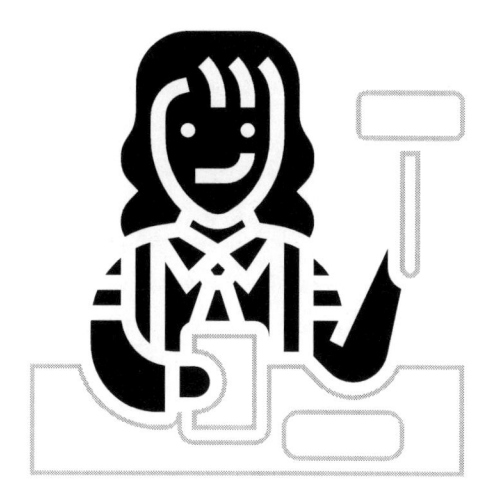

The Verdict!

A bunch of you might read this and say, "The clear-cut winner has to be clean fasting. I mean, Laurel lost a pound more."

Well, I'm here to tell you that this theory isn't complete. When asked after the two months-long fast, Jeannie said that even though her loss was slightly less, she would not give up the fast for anything. The funny thing is that her loss wasn't less, and neither was it more. This exercise that both women went on was the perfect example of how fasting is different for different people. The key thing to note however is that there is no a clear-cut way of fasting.

These two methods were effective for the people who did them. They went on similar journeys and the main mistake that was made was the fact that they spent so much time comparing when they could have just focused on

INTERMITTENT FASTING

what they had to do. Laurel's clean fasting was more tailored to her, and while Jeannie would have also benefited from clean fasting, she wouldn't have gotten the extra benefits that she had gotten when she decided that dirty fasting was the one for her. The same could be said for Laurel and dirty fasting.

In the end, these are two reasonably working methods that people should pick when they know what they want. That is why preparation is one of the first steps in getting ready for a fast. You need to do the research required to know what is going to be beneficial for you. That way you will be better equipped to make a choice and it will be the right one.

Part

04

Tips & Tricks
Just For You!

CHAPTER - 09

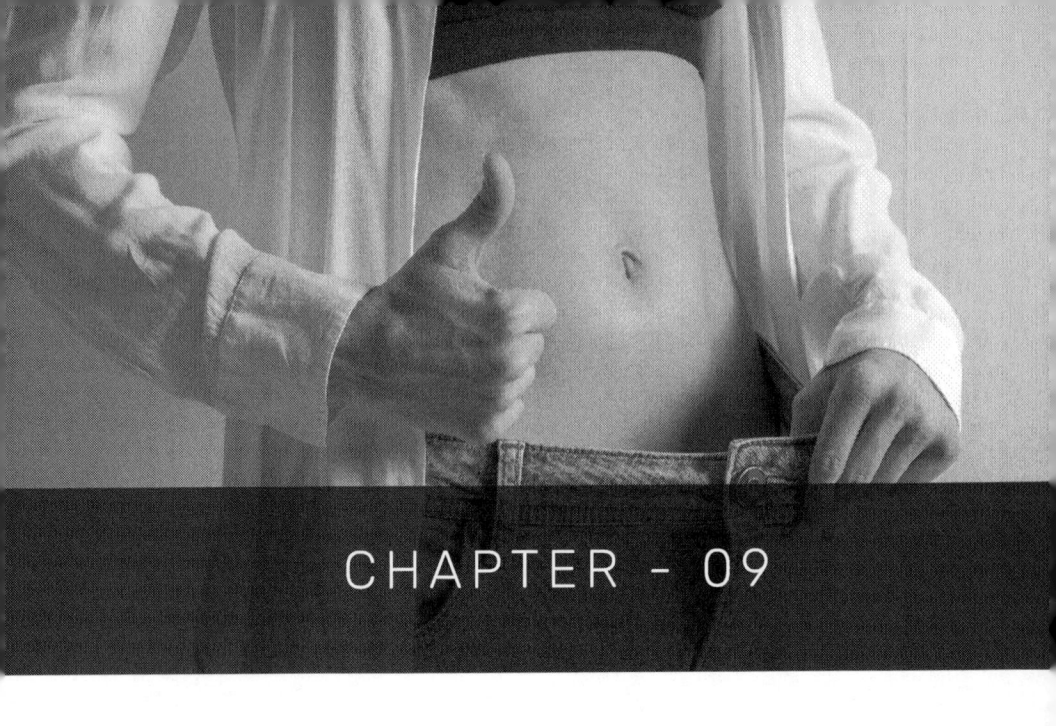

Why is Consistency and Physical Exercises are important in your Weight-Loss Journey?

Being consistent in everything is important. The way our bodies function, they need to be constantly doing something for them to get used to it, and this applies to each and every part of our lives. From the way we talk and use specific patterns of speech, to the way we act and move. If you go to a place many times, after a while, your body gets used to it and you could even do that with your eyes closed.

INTERMITTENT FASTING

This is the same for exercise. You start with a few reps of a particular exercise and soon your body gets used to it and you find it easy to do.

When you put a pattern on repeat, it not only boosts your motivation, but also spontaneity. Here is the correct mix for maximum results and no boredom.

Consistency is by far one of the most important and powerful tools you can have. "Your brain craves it," Andrew Deutscher, who is the M.D. of the Energy Project, which is performance-improvement research and consulting firm, says that your brain craves consistency. Consistency does not just power you through your daily activities so you can achieve what you set out for yourself, but also makes hard routines feel automatic, and that way you'll stay motivated.

However, when you rely on consistency alone, it can get dull. Sometimes, what you need are spontaneous experiences that can add a bit of novelty to keep you engaged. These tap into the reward center in your brain, thereby providing you with hits of pleasure and as a result you feel refreshed and inspired.

The question now is this, how do you stay consistent and yet unconstrained at the same time? There is an answer and it is the key to success! The following techniques will help you create a balance between being ready and steady for anything.

1. DIG WITHIN YOURSELF

You need to start with a strong base to achieve consistency before you can throw spontaneity into the mix. For those healthy things to stick to you, you need to identify a higher reason for them. That reason will then give you all the psychological pushes that you need to pull through. Let's say you are trying to do some workouts at 6:00 a.m. for three days a week. You must make a list of all the meaningful reasons why you must get going and to come up with these reasons, consider the following;

INTERMITTENT FASTING

How will the exercise routine improve your life? For example, if spending a lot more time with your friends is important for you to do, then an exercise routine in the morning can help you free up the evenings and that way you can have your get-togethers. So, when your brain starts to think up excuses, you will have a ready reply that will help you to move forward.

2. GIVE YOURSELF A LITTLE WIGGLE ROOM

Once you have gotten into the groove with your new routine, you must then allow yourself to have the possibility of deviation from it when necessary. If not, without any wiggle room, the smallest disturbance can make you feel like a failure. When you have given yourself some space to move, this increases your overall dedication. That is what the Journal of Consumer Psychology says and therefore you should plan these things ahead. Expect that things could happen to the schedule that you have created and only then will you be able to actively prepare if something actually occurs.

You should have an alternative plan, like a plan B that you go to when dinner invites come in that might throw off the eating routine, you are on (such as choosing to treat yourself to the dinner as a reward and maybe eating a healthy and light breakfast in the morning). This allows you to embrace interruptions and see them as happy surprises. If you follow these tips, then you will stay consistent and avoid being in a rut.

3. KNOW WHEN TO QUIT

Consistency can make you blaze through some challenging routines without even thinking about it at all which is a great thing, but it can make you also stay true to a formula or pattern that you have outgrown. That is why you need to enjoy the comfort and safety of a routine, of course, but you also need to keep an eye on what your results tell you so that you know when it is time to make

INTERMITTENT FASTING

some much-needed changes. Check with yourself at least once a month. You must think about all the progress you have made in your recent efforts and then focus on what your next steps will be. If the benefits of what you are currently doing look like they are fading then you need to take another look at your routine and see what needs adding or subtracting for fresh benefits.

In conclusion, consistency will go a long way in helping you achieve your goals, but you need to understand that you cannot just laze around in it, because by doing so, you can never move forward. All you will be is someone consistent in their stagnation.

Allow yourself room to grow, and if it gets too hard for you, try to be consistent in that until you can surpass it as well. I can promise you that your journey to weight loss will not be the same after that.

There are times where it doesn't seem like you are making any progress, but all you need to do is trust the process and follow it diligently. In no time, you will exceed what you are currently doing and you will break far past those limits.

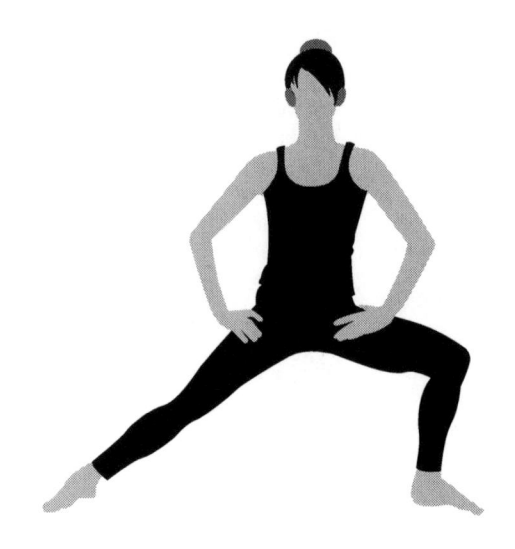

Physical Exercises

We all need a bit of help. These are a few things that are basically a guarantee that you will reach the goal that you want. All you have to do is pick out what you think will work for you and create a routine. From the numerous number of exercises outlined below, for sure there is one for everyone. Based on what you've read so far, all you need to do is find the pattern that is consistent with you and hopefully these tips and tricks will be of great help to you as well as give you the desired results.

These exercises and recipes can to be followed directly but do not neglect to contact your doctor to see if any of these exercises or recipes are things that you can do because of your medical state.

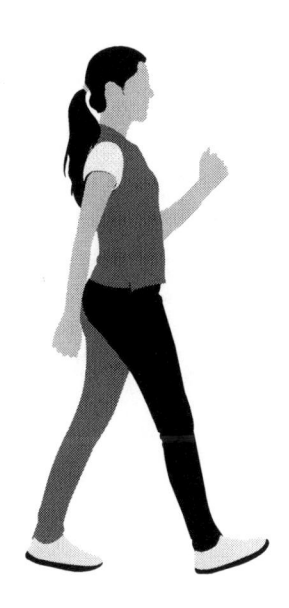

Exercise Suitable for Women Over 40 years

We have talked about fasting in general and we have also discussed intermittent fasting at length. These all give internal developments benefits like better blood nutrient levels and better circulation. They also give external developments too and a perfect example of this is weight loss.

However, if you want to get the most out of intermittent fasting, or you just want to get fit in general, you can try out the following exercises.

INTERMITTENT FASTING

— **MEDITATION**

We're starting with one of the most popular and less strenuous forms of exercise; meditation. When you decide to meditate, what happens is that the information overload which builds up in you from day to day and in turn contributes to your stress is cleared. It has so many benefits, including emotional and health benefits.

The emotional benefits that you can get from meditation often include the following;

- It helps you gain new perspectives on situations that are stressful.
- It helps you build skills that in turn manage stress.
- Your self-awareness increases.
- You are more drawn to focus on current situations.
- Negative emotions are reduced.
- There is a boost in your imagination.
- Your creativity increases as well.
- You learn patience and tolerance from guided meditation.

The effects of meditation on illnesses have also been researched extensively. Meditation is very useful when there is a medical condition present and this has an added effect, especially when the medical condition is stress-related.

While there is a growing body of research to support the health benefits of meditation scientifically, some researchers have also not been able to make valid conclusions about what the possible health benefits of meditation might be.

With this in mind, there is still some research that suggests meditation can be of help to people with the below conditions, in the management of symptoms;

INTERMITTENT FASTING

- Depression.
- Chronic pain.
- Anxiety.
- Cancer.
- Chronic pain.
- Asthma.
- Heart disease.
- Tension headaches.
- High blood pressure.
- Sleep problems.
- Irritable bowel syndrome.

However, make sure to talk to your doctor about the pros and the cons that come with using meditation, especially if you have or possess any of the conditions or health problems listed above.

It is important to note that Meditation should not be used or considered as a replacement for the actual medical treatment, . although it is a useful addition to your other activities like intermittent fasting.

TYPES OF MEDITATION

- Mantra meditation.
- Guided meditation.
- Mindfulness meditation.
- Tai chi.
- Qi gong.

INTERMITTENT FASTING

— DOING YOGA

If you have ever done a downward dog yoga position, you can attest to feeling a lot more relaxed than before. Your level of expertise when it comes to yoga doesn't even matter. As long as you are practicing regularly, then you will feel better throughout your body.

Yoga gives you mental and physical health benefits and this is important especially at this age. If you have an illness, or you are recovering from surgery, or even if you are living some sort of chronic condition, then yoga can become one of the most important parts of your treatment and it could also hasten your healing.

The benefits of yoga include;

Improved strength, flexibility and balance.

> Deep breathing exercises and slow movements help to increase your blood flow while helping you warm up your muscles. Holding a pose could help build your strength.

It can help with spinal pain.

> Yoga is a good use of basic stretching to ease your pain and also improve the mobility of those with pain in their lower back. The American College of Physicians had also recommended yoga as one of the first-line treatments of chronic lower back pain.

It eases the symptoms of arthritis.

> Yoga has been proven to be a way to ease the discomfort of swollen joints for those with arthritis. This is according to Johns Hopkins' review of almost a dozen recent studies.

INTERMITTENT FASTING

It helps with heart health.

Regularized yoga practices may help in reducing the levels of stress and other things that may contribute to having healthier hearts. Several factors that contribute to heart disease, which include excess weight and high blood pressure can be helped through yoga.

It relaxes you and also helps you to sleep better.

Research has shown that a consistent yoga routine before bed can help get you in a ready mindset that helps your body get to sleep and sleep well.

It can cause brighter moods and gives more energy.

Doing yoga is known to increase a person's physical and even mental energy. This is added to a boost in enthusiasm and alertness. There are fewer feelings of negativity after getting a routine of yoga practice.

It helps you manage stress better.

The National Institutes of Health has put forth scientific evidence that shows how yoga supports mental health, stress management, weight loss, healthy eating, and quality sleep.

It helps to connect you to a supportive community.

Going to yoga classes can help you curb feelings of loneliness and also help to provide a safe environment for group support and healing. Even one-on-one sessions can reduce loneliness.

INTERMITTENT FASTING

Yoga poses to try:

- Downward Dog Pose
- Corpse Pose (Savasana)
- Cat-Cow Pose
- Tree Pose
- Child Pose
- Mountain Pose
- Legs-Up-the-Wall Pose

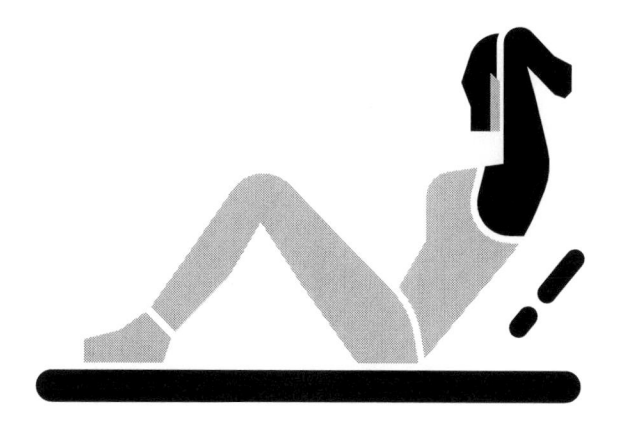

4 Easy Home Workouts to Burn Fat

After the exercises that have been listed out, a few more should be added. These are exercises that have been known to help with weight loss and good health in general. Most of these are everyday exercises, but they will require you to have time on your hands to work out, that is why they aren't necessarily listed with those above. Remember, consistency is the key to exercise and as you take these up, keep at it, and in no time, they will get a lot easier for you to do them.

PLANKS

We have all heard of some variation of this exercise. It is one of the most commonly done exercises that fit into a lot of routines. Here, you go down to the floor, belly down. Then you lift up your weight until your elbows (which should be moved to the side and then you raise your entire body. From here it is supported by your arms and your feet. For a beginner, you could start by putting your knees on the floor, and then when you get the hang of this, you can lift your knees for the added effect.

The benefits of this exercise are tremendous. It's one of the few exercises that can target many places at once. Your arms and legs get toned, and your glutes get their work out as well, and the amount of core strength from this is massive. For a start, you could try the 45-days plank challenge. This starts with a small 10-second plank on your first day and then an added 10 seconds every day and even before the end of those 45 days, you'll see a major difference.

— SQUATS

There is a very high chance that every single person reading this book has done squats before. It requires very little to execute and yet, it brings great results. This exercise targets your glutes and legs, giving them strength and it's quite easy to do.

To execute this, you stand up straight with the tip of both your feet pointing forwards. Next, you put out your hands like you're getting ready to push a wall in front of you. Next, you bend at the knees, while trying your best to keep your back straight. Squat down to a point where your thighs are horizontal and then come back to the starting position. You can do this with weights for added effects.

Increased repetition bring increased results, but should try to pace yourself. It is more important that this exercise is done correctly, than "how many" squats you're able to do. You could do a hundred squats and get nothing out of them if you aren't doing it properly.

INTERMITTENT FASTING

LUNGES

Like the squats, lunges are great because they involve repeated movements. Lunges work all major leg muscles, especially those that are involved in walking. It is quite common to feel a level of freedom in leg movement if lunges are part of your daily routine and they are also easy to do.

To execute this; first, you stand in a position similar to those of the squats. Your feet should face forward and your back should be straight. Now the difference is that you can either put your hands forward like in the squats or keep them on your waist, although it is more common for your hands to be on your waist. Next, you put one leg forward and you bend on it, keeping the knee joint at a 90-degree angle. As your weight comes down on it, you bring it back to your starting position, and then you do the same thing, but with your other leg. You do this in alternation with each other.

ABDOMINAL CRUNCHES

So, you've been on the intermittent fasting diet for a while and you are also starting to notice the change it comes with. Now your next thing is to target your abdomen to help make it firmer. Few exercises do this as well as the abdominal crunches. Unlike sit-ups that involve a few more muscles, these involve only the abdominal muscles, hence its effect is greater. The good thing about this as well is that there are a lot of variations to choose from, but we will be straight with the classical type.

First, lie with your back flat on the floor or exercise matt. Pull your knees towards you, and give your feet a bit of space. Next, put your hands behind your head as support. Breathe out and lift your upper body to your knees, then breathe in and return to your starting position.

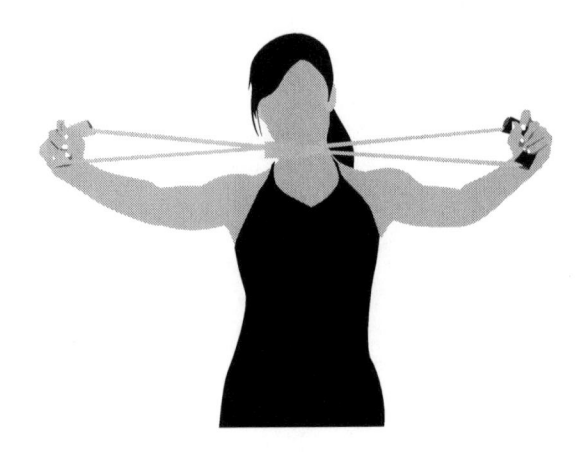

Converting Outdoor Activities to Physical Exercises

The two exercises mentioned above are probably the most important ones, but there are also other exercises to try.

WALKING/JOGGING

Walking or jogging will to go a long way in keeping you healthy. The added mobility helps your joints and the constant movement supports circulation, leading to better heart health. The benefits are endless and consistency in this is key. Therefore, find a little bit of time to go jogging or for long walks once in a while.

INTERMITTENT FASTING

SWIMMING

Occasionally swimming, or participating in water exercises is also good to keep you fit and healthy. When this is combined with intermittent fasting, the benefits are astronomical.

INTERMITTENT FASTING

5 Healthy Diet Recipes you must TRY!

Certain things need to be added to intermittent fasting for it to function at its most optimum. These can range from subtle changes in routine to dietary intake. This sectional will give you five best recipes that are sure to help when combined with intermittent fasting.

Chicken Stir-Fry

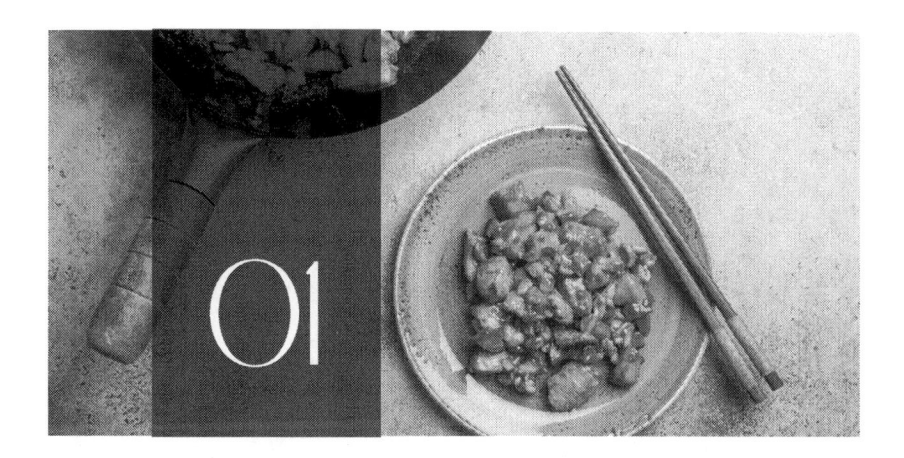

Chicken stir fry is already such a popular and common meal. This recipe is a healthier version to help with minimizing the calories you will have to consume.

INGREDIENTS

- 800ml of chicken stock
- 400g of skinless chicken breasts
- 200g of dried soba noodles
- 2 tbsp of rapeseed oil
- a thumb-sized piece of ginger (grated)
- 2 cloves of garlic (crushed)
- ½ red chili (seeds removed and finely diced)
- 1 red onion (sliced thinly)
- 1 carrot (peeled and shredded)
- 150g of green beans (trimmed)

INTERMITTENT FASTING

- 150g of chestnut mushrooms (sliced)
- 1½ tbsp of low-sodium soy sauce
- 1 tsp of toasted sesame oil
- ½ coriander (a small bunch and roughly chopped)

PREPARATION

Set the stock to a simmer inside a wide and deep pan, placed over medium to low heat. Next add the chicken, ensuring that it is completely submerged. Cook this for about 20 minutes or so, or until it is cooked through. Then remove the chicken but leave the stock in the pan. Next shred the chicken and then set it aside.

Add your noodles to the pan with the stock and then simmer for 3 to 4 minutes or until it is cooked. Drain it, reserving 100ml of the stock. Put the noodles aside.

In a large frying pan or wok, heat the oil. Stir-fry the garlic, chili, and ginger for just 30 seconds. Add in the carrot, onions, mushrooms, and beans and stir-fry for 4 to 6 minutes. Next, add the noodles, shredded chicken, soy, sesame oil, and about half of the reserved stock into the pan. Add a bit more stock if the noodles seem too dry. Divide this between serving plates and then serve with the coriander scattered on.

INTERMITTENT FASTING

02

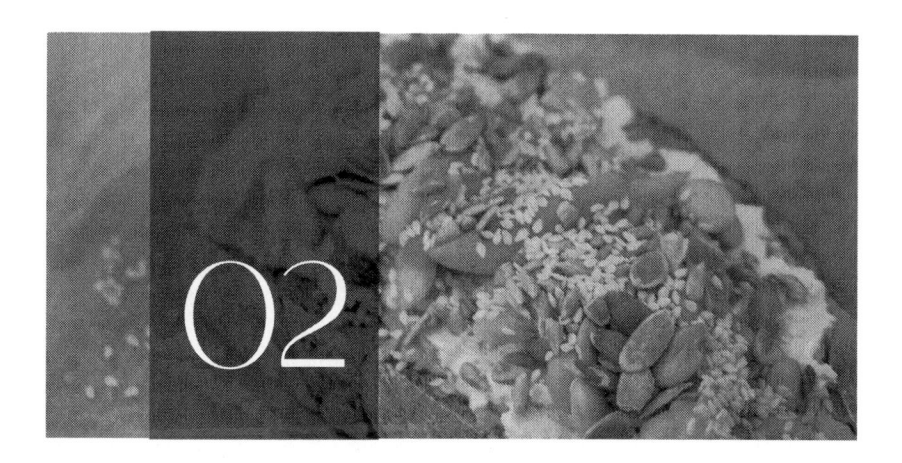

Broad Beans On Toast

If you don't like the normal version of this popular dish, then here's a greener and healthier version that you're sure to enjoy. It's a quick and easy breakfast recipe to help you out as you start the day, especially if your fasting involves a meal plan that lets you eat in the morning. If it does then this is what would be perfect to give you the energy to pull through the fasting period.

INGREDIENTS

- 300g of broad beans (blanched and double-podded)
- A handful of rockets
- 1 clove of garlic
- 30g of pecorino or vegetarian alternative (with extra to serve)
- ½ of a lemon (zested and juiced)
- 75ml of extra-virgin olive oil
- 6 slices of sourdough (toasted)
- A pinch of chili flakes (optional)

INTERMITTENT FASTING

PREPARATION

- Using a food processor, grind a quarter of the broad beans, grind all of the garlic, rocket, lemon, and juice, and the pecorino with some olive oil and seasoning. Add the rest of the broad beans and pulse just a few times. That leaves it chunky.
- Using a spoon, put this on the toast. Next, sprinkle with chili flakes, and then just a drizzle of olive oil and you are good to go.

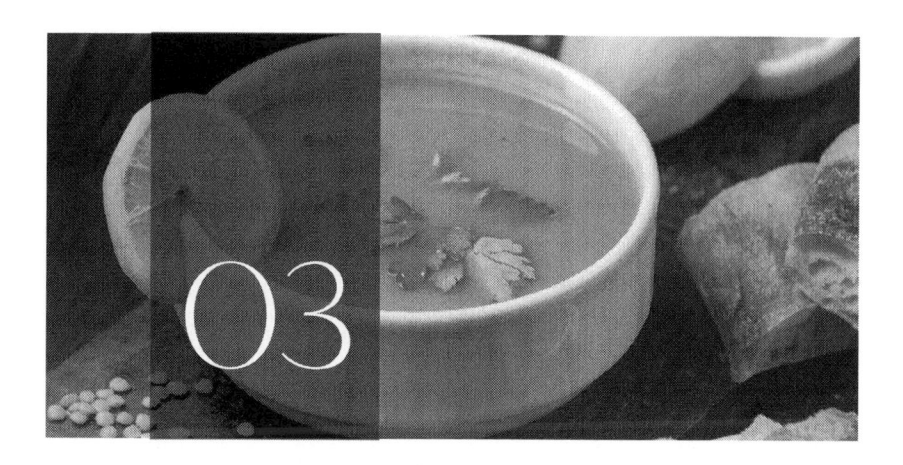

Carrots and Lentil Soup

Next is a simple soup that is easily accessible and very easy to make. It helps with maintaining your calorie intake and is very convenient. This is also an alternative for solid meals.

INGREDIENTS

- 2 tbsp of groundnut oil
- 2 onions (diced)
- 500g of carrots (diced)
- 1 tbsp of mild curry powder
- 4 tbsp of red lentils
- 1.5 liters of vegetable stock
- 1 tsp of cumin seeds
- 4 tbsp of either natural yogurt or coconut yogurt
- A small bunch of coriander (leaves picked)

INTERMITTENT FASTING

PREPARATION

- Heat a tablespoon of vegetable oil in a pan and then soften the carrots and onions for about 10 minutes. Add the curry powder next and fry for just 2 minutes before you add the stock and lentils. Let this simmer and boil for the next 20 minutes until both the carrots and lentils are tender and soft. Season it with pepper and add a little salt if needed.
- Take the pan off the heat and pour it into a stick blender. Blend until it is smooth (you could also blend in a food processor before pouring it back into the pan for reheating).
- Heat the rest of your vegetable oil in a frying pan, then add the cumin seeds until they are golden and fragrant.
- Fill each soup bowl with a spoonful of yogurt. Next, add the cumin seeds and just a sprinkle of coriander leaves.

INTERMITTENT FASTING

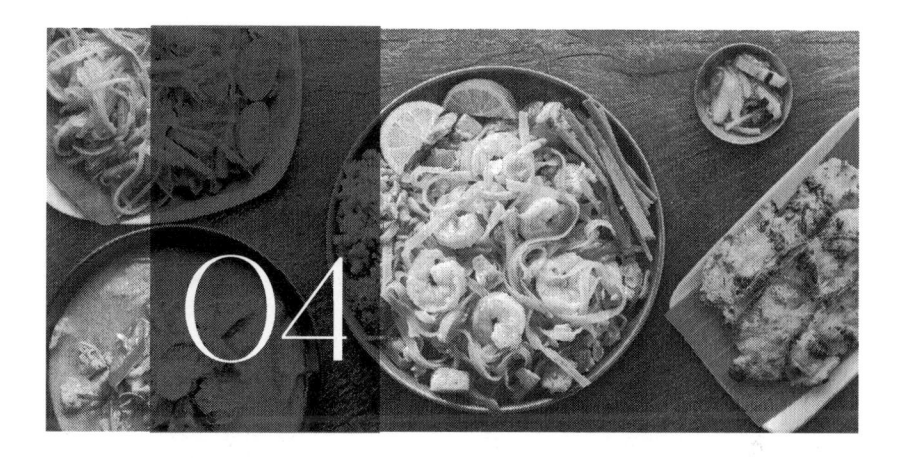

PAD-THAI

And here we have the recipe for a much healthier and lighter pad Thai. It is a great addition to whatever fats you decide on, as it pairs well with the energy requirements.

INGREDIENTS

- Some sesame oils
- 1 red chili (diced)
- 1 tbsp of grated ginger
- 1 clove of garlic (crushed)
- 2 spring onions (sliced)
- 1 egg (beaten with a bit of seasoning)
- 1 mooli (shredded or spiralized)
- 2 courgettes, (shredded or spiralized)
- 50g of bean sprouts

INTERMITTENT FASTING

- 200g of cooked and peeled prawns
- 1 lime (juiced)
- 1 tbsp of fish sauce
- ½ a bunch of coriander (chopped)
- 2 tbsp of roasted peanuts (chopped)

PREPARATION

Heat a tablespoon of sesame oil in a wok until it is very hot. Stir fry the ginger, chili, and garlic until they are fragrant. Next, add the spring onions but for only a few minutes before you scrape everything to one side of the wok. Now add the egg. Swiftly stir-fry this mixture and toss everything all around in the wok. This is to get the scrambled eggs mixed in with the chili and the spring onions. Toss it in the courgette noodles and molly, and stir-fry for about 4 minutes. Next, add in your bean sprouts and prawns. Cook this mixture for another 3 minutes until you are sure the prawns have been warmed through and the water from the vegetable oil has evaporated. Next, add the juice from the lime and the fish sauce. Lastly, scatter this with the chopped peanuts and coriander to serve.

INTERMITTENT FASTING

05

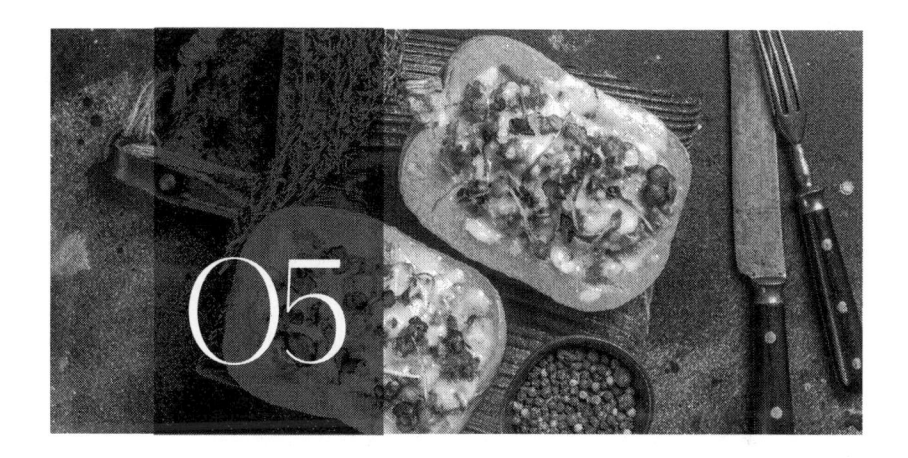

Stuff Butternut Squash with Feta

This is a vegetarian meal. A lot of people do not incorporate fruits elements in their meals, so this should be a healthy change, and a delicious one too.

INGREDIENTS

- 1 butternut squash (large)
- 2 tbsp of olive oil
- 2 long shallots (diced)
- 2 cloves of garlic (crushed)
- 200g of basmati rice
- 400ml of vegetable stock
- 1 lemon (zested and juiced)
- 4 tbsp of raisins or dried cranberries
- ½ small bunch of oregano leaves (picked and chopped)
- ½ small bunch of dill (chopped)

INTERMITTENT FASTING

- 2 tbsp of pine nuts (toasted)
- 100g of feta
- 320g of winter greens or spinach (steamed)

PREPARATION

- First, preheat the oven to 200°C. Then cut your squash in half, and using a spoon, remove the seeds. Rub with half of the oil, season it, and put it on a baking tray with the cut side facing up. Roast this for 40 minutes.
- While this happens, heat the rest of the oil in a medium-sized pan. Fry up the shallots for about 10 minutes until they are soft. Then you add the garlic, fry for about 30 seconds, and then add the rice too and cook this for 2 minutes, while stirring so that you coat it in the shallots and the oil.
- Pour in the lemon zest, vegetable stock, and lemon juice, then bring it to a simmer. Next, stir in the raisins, add most of the herbs but not all the pine nuts. Turn heat to medium or low and cover it. Cook this for 12-15 minutes. This should be enough time for the rice to get tender and for the stock to be absorbed.
- After about 40 minutes, you need to bring out the squash from the oven. Next, use a spoon and scoop out some of the flesh in the center to create a hollow (you can chop and stir the flesh before adding it into any rice that is leftover or you can use it in another recipe).
- Fluff your rice with a fork. After that, use a spoon to dig into the hollowed-out center of the squash. Crumble the feta into this. Turn the oven up to about 220°C and then bake the halves of the squash for about 10 minutes until the feta on top is crisp and golden. Scatter the remaining herbs and pine nuts on this, and serve along with any rice that remains. Serve with wilted spinach or winter greens.

part

05

The Proven Weight-Loss Journey

CHAPTER - 10

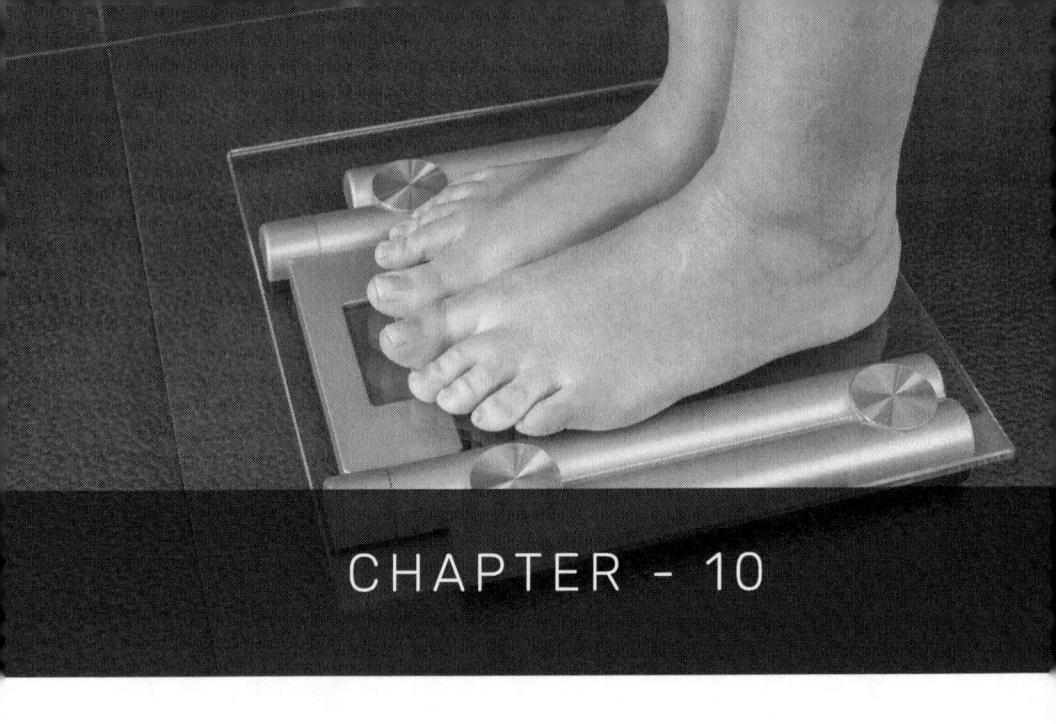

Real-Life Weight Loss Experience for Women over 40 years through Intermittent Fasting

I feel like an important part of intermittent fasting is knowing that you are definitely not the only one taking it. Thousands of people around the world fast every day, and although it may be for different reasons, you should know that there are people at another end of the globe who are reading this book at the same time as you. They too are thinking about starting their weight loss journey with intermittent fasting. That should be seen as a sense of comfort, that people around the world are going through the things you are going through, and it is an assurance that you are not alone.

INTERMITTENT FASTING

With that in mind, it's not just people who are about to start intermittent fasting that should be considered. I feel it is just as important for you to hear from people who have already gone on this journey and have come out with results that they never thought they would be able to get. This should be enough in terms of motivation that can get you started.

MIRA, 41

I decided to starve myself before my wedding to fit into the dress. I was going to do this for a month because I was already very overweight, bordering on obesity. I just wanted something that would help me shed a few pounds before the greatest day of my life, and since nothing else worked for me, I chose to go without food. I was already on this when one of my bridesmaids told me to just try intermittent fasting instead of flat out starving myself. I had no idea what it meant at the time, but she planned out the entire thing for me and told me exactly what I needed to do and when. A month came and I had to even sit down my dress a bit because the weight loss was tremendous. I couldn't stop after that. I continued intermittent fasting for a whole year and I'm down more than 30 pounds and still keeping it consistent.

KATHY, 39

I have practiced law for over 13 years. When I lost my first major case, it sent me into a deep depression that took months of therapy to pull me out of. By the time I was out, I had completely let myself go. I had been able to get my confidence back to some extent, but I had never been able to regain my figure. The sad part was that I couldn't start exercising. I wanted to, but I was not afforded the time. I didn't see the point of using the little vacation time I had to exercise as well. It

INTERMITTENT FASTING

was meant for relaxation and letting go, and that was all I wanted to do. Still, because my weight went unchecked, I continued to grow and grow until it was too uncomfortable for me to stand there on the court in front of the judge and the jury and not feel like my weight was a factor. In one of my cases, I had to do a bit of research on fasting and that's when I came across intermittent fasting. It stuck instantly and I started to practice it. I have practiced it faithfully for the past four years and on the 6th of February, 2021, I recorded my official loss of a total of 100 pounds.

DENISE, 46

With my only daughter headed for college, I had more time to myself. I decided to try out something new. I had heard about intermittent fasting in an article online, while I was trying to make a meal plan for my daughter. We both came to the consensus that we would do it together; me while I was here and she, while she was at college. Her case was more along the lines of solidarity because I was the one who was overweight.

I tried it for a month, and I won't lie, it was half-assed. I didn't see any major changes, but my daughter did. She told me things like she was able to focus more and felt more confident about herself. I couldn't believe that it was the same thing that I did. So, I continued for the next few months, and this time, I followed my schedule to the letter, and now, here I am with a figure that rivals what I was in my twenties. I even feel as good as I did back then.

INTERMITTENT FASTING

6 Celebrities Who Practice Intermittent Fasting

According to: The Medium & Marie Claire

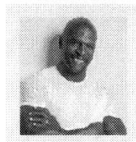

TERRY CREWS
The famous *Brooklyn Nine-Nine Actor*, ex-professional football player, comedian, and health enthusiast.

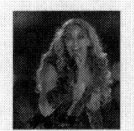

BEYONCE
The Queen of Destiny's Child, the legendary American singer-songwriter

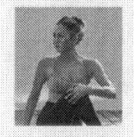

JENNIFER ANISTON
American actress, producer, and businesswoman who rose to fame in the show *F.R.I.E.N.D.S* playing the role of Rachel Greene.

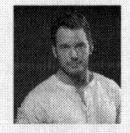

CHRIS PRATT
Famous actor, comedian, and widely known for his roles in *'Guardians of the Galaxy'* and *'Jurassic World'*

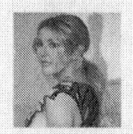

ELLIE GOULDING
English singer-songwriter and record producer who is popular with her song *'Love Me Like You Do'*

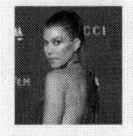

KOURTNEY KARDASHIAN
The famous American media personality, model, and socialite.
According to: *The Medium - The Fasting Secrets by Tim Marie Claire Australia*

THE PROVEN WEIGHT-LOSS JOURNEY

The Author's Point of View

INTERMITTENT FASTING

You could say that this book is the fulfillment of a personal dream for me. The fact that I can help so many people on their way to a new chapter of their lives is something that is unbelievably satisfying. This isn't just some gathered talk, you can take this from me since I've had my own experience with intermittent fasting.

Intermittent fasting, as I've mentioned before, is not a new concept to the world, but just like you, it was a new concept to me at a certain point in my life. Like most of you, I could not imagine why I should starve myself because I wanted to get healthy. By my definition, food was healthy, so all I needed to do was try to keep eating healthy but in time, I came to realize that it's not always enough. Healthy eating is important and that is an undisputed fact, but in reality, how often can we keep up such a lifestyle?

Healthy eating alone requires special planning and preparation, but more often than not, we don't have the luxury it takes to do this. In this way, intermittent fasting sort of helps us with balancing this because we don't have to plan and prepare meals as often. Instead, we can do this at our convenience, after we have picked doubt the intermittent fasting technique that best suits our schedule.

On top of all of these, there is still the added option of ordering healthy food. There are companies and delivery services that specialize in providing healthy meals in appropriate proportions. They can be planned out and picked based on what would work best for you.

I discovered these things personally when I started my journey, and I remember wishing there was an all-encompassing guide, just like this one that would teach me what I needed to know. Sure, you could probably see articles here and there, trying to help, or helpful videos online, but the sad reality is that you would probably have to go through dozens of them, or even more before you can find the answers to what you want to know.

INTERMITTENT FASTING

I suffered the same fate, and I couldn't believe it. It made me feel like this was not something that people took seriously. I decided to compile my own data, little by little, just to see where it went. I started my intermittent fasting journey with the knowledge I had searched for and after a while, (it wasn't even a long time) I started to see amazing results.

I was dumbfounded! Something I had decided to try only as a test run, had started to change my life. I felt lighter, my repeated days of feeling bloated were long behind me. I was energetic and more importantly, I had lost tremendous amounts of weight. I knew that I couldn't be the only one who could testify to this. So, just like I was known to do, I did the research. I found hundreds of people online who were happy to share their stories of intermittent fasting and how it worked for them.

Most of them, like me, had decided to just give it a try, and when the results began to show, they had eventually continued and soon it had become a lifestyle choice. These were people from different walks of life, even celebrities were vocal about how intermittent fasting helped them even with their disastrously busy schedules.

That was when I decided to create this guide, for people who want to try this intermittent fasting but are scared to do something uncertain. This book will help curb those fears, by giving you facts, research, and testimonies from people who have done what you are about to try.

Why? Because I believe in the power of intermittent fasting. I know first-hand how effective it is and all that you need to add to it are things that are well explained in this text.

On your weight loss journey, you've hit a gold mine, just like me. It only has to be done right, and best of all; intermittent fasting can fit into almost any schedule you have. There are only a few cases where it is discouraged and those cases are even listed here, to save you the trouble it takes of doing the amount of research it requires to find things like that. I do not doubt that you saw some questions that did not occur to you at first, but they made a lot of sense when you read them. That is exactly my aim, to bring this information right to you. I do this because I completely believe that intermittent fasting works!

Conclusion

INTERMITTENT FASTING

This book was made as a guide to a specific demographic, but I do not doubt that it will be helpful to other many people as well.

You can think of this as all of us, you and I and millions of people around the world, going on a journey together and at least that journey has reached its end. But I hope that in the end, the knowledge that you have gotten from this book will be a constant companion as I welcome you to this wonderful new lifestyle that should be a thrilling ride for you.

The long-standing history of fasting is fascinating, as you've seen, with the numerous famous characters who boasted of its legacy, using their lives as a testament to what it could do. As you have read this book and you go on your journey, I wish you the same success that they had and even more.

It's now our turn to carry on the legacy and soon, we will be the ones whose testimonies people would read off and make the choice for a healthier body and mind overall.

It is up to us to make sure that we live in a healthy and more energetic world. The only way to do this is if we, our loved ones, and everyone else around us can be healthy, and now that you have unlocked the key to good health and vitality, I need you to share this with those who you care for and love. They too deserve to be part of this achievement.

Intermittent fasting is a healthy lifestyle choice for you and as long as you are willing, you will see great results in no time. The best part, as we have said many times, is how it spills into other areas of your life and affects them positively too.

Remember that you have to be consistent. The lack of consistency will ruin you and your progress therefore you need to keep at it, for as long as it takes. Keep track of how well you are doing, and then add to that and try again. You will grow and succeed.

INTERMITTENT FASTING

Congratulations on your move to want to lose weight, live healthily and feel better. I will see you at the other end of this trip when you feel a lot lighter and better than you have ever felt. You can tell your friends and loved ones about this new technique that you have learned from this book. Again, congratulations and good luck in everything you do!

References

INTERMITTENT FASTING

Gunnars K, (2020): Intermittent Fasting 101 – *The Ultimate Beginner's Guide*. Healthline
https://www.healthline.com/nutrition/intermittent-fasting-guide

Diet Review: *Intermittent Fasting for Weight Loss*. The Nutrition Source
https://www.hsph.harvard.edu/nutritionsource/healthy-weight/diet-reviews/intermittent-fasting/

Gunnars, K (2021): *10 Evidence-Based Health Benefits of Intermittent Fasting*. Healthline
https://www.healthline.com/nutrition/10-health-benefits-of-intermittent-fastingv

Bubnoff, AV (2021): The when of eating: The science behind intermittent fasting. Knowable Magazine
https://knowablemagazine.org/article/health-disease/2021/the-when-eating-update-intermittent-fasting

Rowan, A (2021): Intermittent fasting, its health benefits for you, and weight loss without the calorie counting. SCMP Lifestyle / Health & Wellness
https://www.scmp.com/lifestyle/health-wellness/article/3136902/intermittent-fasting-its-health-benefits-you-and-weight

Tello, M, MD, MPH (2020): *Intermittent Fasting: Surprising Update*. Harvard Health Publishing
https://www.health.harvard.edu/blog/intermittent-fasting-surprising-update-2018062914156

Romero. T. (2021): *Thinking of trying Intermittent Fasting?* A healthy Philly.
https://www.phillyvoice.com/intermittent-fasting-benefits-16-8-weight-loss-diets/

INTERMITTENT FASTING

Gleeson, JR (2019): Intermittent Fasting: *Is it right for you?* Michigan Health. https://healthblog.uofmhealth.org/wellness-prevention/intermittent-fasting-it-right-for-you

Saleeh, N, MD. MS (2019): *8 Reasons Why Most Diet Fails, According to A health expert.* MDLinx https://www.mdlinx.com/article/8-reasons-why-most-diets-fail-according-to-a-health-expert/3ZkrtxbyazW69yHspaVEDK

Kubala, J., MS, RD (2021): *9 Potential Intermittent Fasting Side Effects.* Healthline https://www.healthline.com/nutrition/intermittent-fasting-side-effects

Torborg, L (2020): Mayo Clinic Q and A. Mayo Clinic https://newsnetwork.mayoclinic.org/discussion/mayo-clinic-q-and-a-long-term-benefits-and-risks

Uttekar, Ps., MD & Allarkha S. MD (2021) *What are the Health Benefits of Fasting?* Medicine Net https://www.medicinenet.com/what_are_the_health_benefits_of_fasting/article.htm

Fasting Secrets by Tim (2020) Medium https://medium.com/@easydifferenceif/celebrities-and-intermittent-fasting-190f189c8ab4

Waterhouse, J. (2020): *9 Celebrities Who Swear by Intermittent Fasting.* Marie Claire https://www.marieclaire.com.au/intermittent-fasting-celebrities

Made in United States
Orlando, FL
05 May 2022